Using the Systems Approach for Aphasia

Using the Systems Approach for Aphasia introduces therapists to systems theory, exploring the way in which a holistic method that is already a key part of other health and social care settings can be employed in aphasia therapy.

Detailed case studies from the author's own extensive experience demonstrate how systemic tools can be incorporated into practice, offering practical suggestions for service delivery and caseload management in frequently overloaded community health services. Exploring the treatment process from first encounters, through the management of goals and attainments, to caring for patients after therapy has ended, the book demonstrates a method of delivering therapy in a way that will better serve the people who live with aphasia and their families, as well as the clinician themselves.

Key features of this book include:

- An accessible overview of systems theory and its use in aphasia therapy.
- Consideration of how current popular ideas such as self-management, holistic rehabilitation and compassion focussed therapy can be incorporated to provide the best treatment.
- Guidance on when and how to involve families based on case studies.
- Case studies throughout to fully illustrate systemic approaches.

An essential resource for both students and seasoned clinicians, the theory explored in this book will provide a fresh approach to therapy and new skills for working with people with aphasia and their families.

Susie Hayden was born and raised in Tanzania; she studied Language and Linguistics at York University, and Postgraduate Speech and Language Therapy in 1990. Susie's passion for working with individuals and families experiencing aphasia, carers and professionals is enhanced by her Systemic Family Therapy training and practice since 2016. An experienced trainer and clinical educator, in both theoretical and practical aspects of aphasia therapy, Susie was Specialist Clinical Advisor to the CQC for four years. After 25 years specialising in aphasia therapy within NHS hospitals and community settings, recent years have seen her focus on charity and voluntary sectors and running her own practice.

First published 2022
by Routledge
2 Park Square, Milton Park, Abingdon, Oxon OX14 4RN

and by Routledge
605 Third Avenue, New York, NY 10158

Routledge is an imprint of the Taylor & Francis Group, an informa business

© 2022 Susie Hayden

British Library Cataloguing-in-Publication Data
A catalogue record for this book is available from the British Library

Library of Congress Cataloging-in-Publication Data
Names: Hayden, Susie, author.
Title: Using the systems approach for aphasia : an introduction for speech and language therapists / Susie Hayden.
Description: Milton Park, Abingdon, Oxon ; New York, NY : Routledge, 2022. | Includes bibliographical references and index.
Identifiers: LCCN 2021025623 (print) | LCCN 2021025624 (ebook) | ISBN 9781032014388 (hardback) | ISBN 9781032014371 (paperback) | ISBN 9781003178613 (ebook)
Subjects: LCSH: Aphasia. | Speech therapist and patient.
Classification: LCC RC425 .H37 2022 (print) | LCC RC425 (ebook) | DDC 616.85/52—dc23
LC record available at https://lccn.loc.gov/2021025623
LC ebook record available at https://lccn.loc.gov/2021025624

ISBN: 978-1-032-01438-8 (hbk)
ISBN: 978-1-032-01437-1 (pbk)
ISBN: 978-1-003-17861-3 (ebk)

DOI: 10.4324/9781003178613

Typeset in Optima
by Apex CoVantage, LLC

Using the Systems Approach for Aphasia

An Introduction for Speech and Language Therapists

Susie Hayden

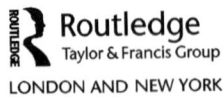

Routledge
Taylor & Francis Group

LONDON AND NEW YORK

Contents

Preface

Aphasia services world-wide are limited and vary enormously in style, level of skill and availability. A systems approach to aphasia therapy embraces the use of systems theory, which is already filtering through to primary health-care and social care settings, to provide a novel way in which to embark on delivery of services for aphasia.

Such an approach unites well-known therapies used in clinics and reha-bilitation settings today, so as to provide the clinician and the student clini-cian with a greater skill set and hence renewed enthusiasm and evidence for their work. More importantly, an adjustment to the balance of power in the clinic affords the person with aphasia and their family a greater sense of agency and hope as they navigate the path towards living successfully with aphasia.

This selection of cases from my own experience of working with aphasia forms the basis of a proposal for systemic tools to be incorporated into the student speech and language therapist experience, as well as that of the practising clinician. The identity of individuals is protected by the use of composite characters.

The unexpected benefits described here support currently popular ideas such as self-management, holistic rehabilitation, compassion focussed ther-apy and Linda Worrall's 'Seven Habits of Highly Effective Aphasia Thera-pists'. Additionally, practice-based evidence for a different approach to aphasia service delivery and caseload management in our frequently over-loaded community health services is described.

It is well known that people with aphasia rarely access mental health support. A new approach to aphasia therapy built upon a systems approach could go a long way to address this in the future. My long-term passion for working with aphasia has been enhanced by adopting a systemic mind-set in my work, which is shared here. I am grateful to those who have taught and continue to teach me so much about the richness of human communication, even in the absence of words. This book is written as much by the many people I have met through my work as by me. It is they who have taught me about courage, survival and the meaning of human communication.

I would like to dedicate this work to the current, past and future members of the Newmarket Aphasia Café, and in loving memory of Dr. Ron Ryall, Emeritus Fellow of Churchill College Cambridge, who fought hard, without success, to improve access to aphasia therapy for himself and others.

Grateful thanks go to all my many teachers mentioned by name in the book. In addition, I am immensely grateful to the ARU family therapy tutors who reignited my interest in aphasia, as well as Enda, Jon and Fi, for reading my proposal and making kind remarks. I am lucky to have a loyal family who encourage me to write. Stephen's proofreading, and his tolerance of having his ear bent are prized; but his kindness and patience are priceless.

Susie Hayden

Notes

1 The words 'client' and 'patient' both feel inadequate terms by which to refer to people I work with as an aphasia therapist, however, in the absence of a better alternative they are both used in the book to refer to the person with aphasia. Throughout the book, the following abbreviations will be used:

PWA = people with aphasia
SLT = speech and language therapist/therapy
OT = occupational therapist

2 'Family' is used throughout the book and it refers to anyone in the close social world of the person with aphasia, not necessarily the traditional family model.

1 | What is systems theory?

The 'systems' view of life is one that has been growing over the last 30 years in a variety of disciplines. It has had major implications for ecology, politics, sociology, sciences, geography, communication and health sciences. A less mechanistic, and more holistic or 'integrative' view is increasingly taken in many fields, and one that unifies all aspects of a problem into a single approach.

Systems theory considers multifactorial elements of a difficulty that presents itself and strives to provide a sustainable solution to problems. Sometimes expressed as 'The whole is more than the sum of its parts', it captures a way of thinking that considers complexity, networks and patterns of organisation in life on earth (Capra and Luisi 2014).

For the purposes of this book, I will be discussing systemic thinking in the context of healthcare and its application in aphasia therapy specifically, although the wider application of this perspective should be borne in mind whilst considering some of the ideas presented here.

Rather than considering, for example, that the body and the mind are separate organisms, a systemic view sees not only the brain but also the immune system, the bodily tissues, and even each cell as a living, cognitive system. 'Evolution is no longer seen as a competitive struggle for existence, but rather as a cooperative dance in which creativity and the constant emergence of novelty are the driving forces' (Capra and Luisi 2014).

Systems theory in healthcare

Honorary professor of public health at the University of Bremen, Helmut Milz, writes 'Modern physicians do not get enough training in understanding illness

DOI: 10.4324/9781003178613-1

1

in context. They are paid for short interventions, which avoid the exploration of emotional issues or anxieties' (Milz 2014). Anne Harrington, a professor of History of Science, explores the history of mind-body medicine in *The Cure Within* (Harrington 2008), and shows that there is increasing evidence for how placebo and nocebo can influence physical recovery and how expectations of recovery and trust in the therapist can lead to better outcomes (Benedetti 2008).

Capra and Luisi (2014) maintain that:

> the basic aim of any therapy will be to restore the patient's balance, and since the underlying model of health acknowledges the organism's innate tendency to heal itself, the therapist will try to intrude only minimally and help create the environment most conducive to the healing. Such an approach to therapy will be multidimensional, involving treatments at several different levels of the mind/body system, which will often require a multidisciplinary team effort. Healthcare of this kind will require many new skills in disciplines not previously associated with medicine and is likely to be intellectually richer, more stimulating and more challenging than a medical practice that adheres exclusively to the biomedical model.

This view is certainly borne out through my own training in systemic family therapy, where I have come to see how systems theory (which is increasingly used in settings such as mental health, social work and the youth justice system), helps to ensure that clients achieve the changes they need, in order to transform their lives.

Family therapies were developed out of systems theory over the course of the 21st century. The anthropologist Gregory Bateson (1904–1980) is often referred to as the 'grandfather' of family therapy; he turned his study of anthropology towards mental health and spent his life exploring systemic approaches to communication, family behaviour and social norms, based on the premise that 'Relationships for human beings are a primary source of existence' (Bateson 1972).

By viewing the context in which the problem or question presents itself, systems theory shows how approaches by which to address such problems might come from a variety of sources. This means that no one approach can be considered to be 'the answer' for every client.

For many health professions, techniques learned during training are designed to be applied to specific sets of circumstances that we encounter. A 'set' case history is taken for every patient, using identical questions. Such a recipe-book approach is of course necessary to some extent: in this way, we create the scaffolding onto which we can hook our learning. Only when we have started this way can we begin to apply more creative approaches to our work and broaden our skill set to meet the individual needs of our clients. In this book, I will be asking whether speech and language therapy students are sufficiently equipped to consider communication impairment in the wider context of the 'systems' to which they and their clients with aphasia belong.

We seem to be constantly striving for the ultimate simple solution in healthcare; the one where an applied formula will solve a range of problems that are presented to us. This can never truly exist when we are dealing with dynamic, complex human beings. With current emphasis on evidence-based practice, there is often a drive to find the latest evidence for therapies, and the assumption that the 'new' is always 'better' than the old. When the 'old' fails to work for us, (only being effective in certain specific circumstances), we immediately discard it in favour of a 'newer' approach. In my use of references from a variety of sources and at different time periods within the last 30 years I hope to demonstrate how we can adopt a more 'joined-up' way of thinking. It is time to consider new ways of thinking about how we understand our clients, ourselves and how a range of aphasia therapies fit into that work. A systems approach combines what we already know and seeks to apply it in different ways.

In some areas of speech and language therapy, there are currently effective prescribed approaches to the treatment of speech disorders, such as LSVT LOUD®, used for dysarthric speech (Ramig et al. 2018). Here, a specific programme will result in good outcomes as shown by research. Having worked for some years as a specialist in voice disorders I am also aware that simple voice techniques can result in dramatic recovery of voice, even after long periods of aphonia. However, for the majority of my experience of a voice caseload, such practical techniques combined with systemic family therapy techniques are the ones that have been the most effective across the board in terms of longer-term outcomes.

Systemic therapy offers professionals invaluable tools with which to offer meaningful change to clients, but importantly, it encourages them to be simultaneously aware of the relationships within their own lives. The therapist is also part of the context of therapy and influences the process (Burnham 2012) as we will see in Chapter 4.

Informed by anthropology, philosophy and Wittgenstein (Biletzki and Matar 2020), developmental psychology, conflict resolution, history, cultural and intercultural and sociological studies, it is by unifying similarities between disciplines as well as embracing differences that sustainable goals can be achieved. The full range of ideas within systemic thinking are extensive and well beyond the scope of this book. Key aspects that have relevance to aphasia therapy will be discussed here.

Social constructionism

Central to the development of systems theory are the ideas of social constructionism and social constructivism (Hoffman 1990). In simplified terms, social constructionism holds the view that we understand the world through a shared understanding with others (for example we all accept rectangles of plastic as constituting a form of currency in our society). What we believe to be true is validated by others. Within a family structure, for example, choices are 'constructed and constrained by inequalities of power and culturally shared discourses' (Dallos and Draper 2010). An example of this might be traditional female roles within the family. Social constructivism, on the other hand, focusses on what an individual understands about the world as a result of their interactions with others. Experiences will be unique for each person.

In the arenas of family functioning and mental health, a systemic approach seeks to understand not only the current affordances and constraints of the context of people's lives, but also how they were in the past and how they might alter in the future. Reflections projected into different timeframes can influence people to alter the way they think about difficulties in the present.

In the past, modernist views within family therapy were around objectivity: science and psychology would be strongly based on observation and controlled experiments, followed up by valid treatments (Gurman and Kniskern 1978). Postmodernism questioned the validity of an objective approach to working with families, as there was so much subjectivity and variability in the views of scientists, as well as within families and between individual family members. The ideas of 'first order' and 'second order' cybernetics were born. This means that family therapies moved way from those more objective, rather 'fixed' ideas, to holding a view that 'reality invariably involves a reconstruction, occurs in relationships and is based on feedback. There is not one accurate view of reality but invariably differing perceptions and constructions' (Dallos and Draper 2010).

Family therapists in Italy in the late 1960s (e.g., Palazzoli, Boscolo, Cecchin and others) began to change the power relationship in keeping with post-modernist social constructionist thinking. This was further influenced by Gregory Bateson, mentioned above. Bateson was anthropologist, social scientist, environmentalist and naturalist:

> He was, in my opinion, one of the most influential thinkers of the 20th century. The uniqueness of his thought came from its broad range and its generality. In an age characterized by fragmentation and overspecialization, Bateson challenged the basic assumptions and methods of several sciences by looking for patterns connecting different phenomena and for processes beneath structures.
>
> (Capra 2018)

Bateson's philosophy of mind and cybernetics described the recursiveness of human interactions (Bateson 1972). This means that when working with an individual or a family, the therapist becomes 'part of the system' they are working in, whilst at the same time trying to maintain a stance of curiosity so as to understand the client and family (Cecchin 1987).

Anderson and Goolishian (1988) stated that 'a problem system is always a linguistic system', and that 'problems do not have an objective existence in and of themselves but only through conversation with others'. This is interesting for me as a linguist who is also a speech and language therapist and reminds us that language does not only reflect what is happening in our lives, but it also creates a view of what is happening; we can alter this view by changing the language we use.

Health professionals will be familiar with terms such as 'an asthmatic', 'an aphasic' or 'a stroke victim'. Such totalising use of language seems to suggest that the injury or 'victimhood' is an inherent part of that individual's identity. These terms may influence how professionals view the future for such individuals or indeed how the person starts to think about their own identity and future. Using more tentative language to describe things opens up the possibility of change for all involved, as we shall see in later case studies.

More recently, in 1992, psychologists Anderson and Goolishian advocated collaborative, reflective and reflexive conversations to create solutions.

They pioneered a 'not knowing' technique that is used to relate to clients within therapy through language and collaboration, and without the use of diagnostic labels. This approach to therapy places the client in control of the therapy session and asks the therapist to focus on the present therapy session and ignore any preconceived notions they may have. Although first developed for the use of family and mental health therapy, it has since expanded into other professional practices such as occupational psychology, higher education and research.

Traditional views of healthcare hold the 'expert' in high esteem, and expect solutions and cures, with the client as a passive recipient. This power is never greater in my view, than when the client who has been deprived of language is facing the therapist or doctor with their full repertoire of words. According to the technique, a 'not knowing' approach to therapeutic conversations is adopted, in order to address the power balance. Preconceptions are shelved; 'Not knowing – our understanding, explanation and interpretation in therapy must not be limited by prior experiences or theoretically formed truths and knowledge' (Anderson and Goolishian 1992).

Barry Mason (1993), a social worker and family therapist, developed his now well established and widely used systemic theory of dealing with risk. He suggested holding 'authoritative doubt' in the presence of a client and their family; personally, I would refer to this as 'suspending one's expertise' in the therapy setting so as to be more open to ideas and to the context of the person in front of you. This will be illustrated in Chapter 5.

Social constructionism brings in linguistic terms, which speech and language therapists with a linguistic background will be familiar with. Postmodern semantics, narrative and linguistics, Noam Chomsky and Ferdinand de Saussure (who founded structural linguistics in 1915) are all part of the systemic story. Previous linguistic theory emphasised the historical development of language, de Saussure added the idea of an organisation of rules for grammar, while Chomsky uncovered the deep structure of what he called transformational grammar. The American sociologist Talcott Parsons, considered one of the most influential figures in sociology in the 20th century, acknowledged the necessity of the 'subjective dimension' of human action in addition to scientific rigour (Parsons 1985). Parsons' discussions took place within the context of systems theory and cybernetics.

Social constructionism listens to the stories of people's lives and sees them through a flexible lens. Things are always in the process of change, and we are always on the way to becoming revised versions of ourselves as we go through our lives, according to what we experience and how we describe that experience. When we listen to a story, we hear it from our own world view and then respond into the world view of the other person; we each operate out of different contexts. What we add and the questions we ask can all shape the way the other person thinks about their story, and recursively, how we think about our own.

Traditional models of therapy

Therapy in the traditional medical model operates from a distance. 'Patients' come to the 'experts' for treatment, and expect to remain relatively passive, until they are better. My observation is that the degree to which individuals feel they are in charge of their recovery varies, not only according to socio-economic status and levels of formal education, but also as a factor of what they have experienced prior to the current situation, medically, socially and psychologically.

Failure to take the treatment or follow advice meted out in the clinic is often met with blame; the client is considered to be and often labelled as 'non-compliant' or 'unmotivated' and sometimes discharged from care as a result. In my experience, such clients often reappear on different caseloads at various times in the future, still 'uncompliant', as their needs have not been met and yet they are still using health resources which would have been better if applied more holistically in the first instance!

One woman reporting some swallowing issues had been told by a neurologist that she did not, as she believed, have MS (multiple sclerosis) but that it was 'only in her head'. A different neurologist said she did have MS and reviewed her annually. This woman kept cropping up on various community caseloads and it was acknowledged that she had somatisation disorder. Eyes rolled and sighs were drawn, as yet again she reported choking on her food, because the experts 'knew' she did not have dysphagia. Her favourite meal was spaghetti on toast, normally quite a challenge for the MS patient. I asked her permission to carry out a full bedside swallowing assessment. I explained how the swallow worked, with diagrams and video clips: together we identified with her what was working well and what was not so good (she did have reduced oral sensation). I acknowledged that her experience was a little different from what I could see. She talked briefly about her personal relationships and I reassured her about her swallowing, offering a telephone or face to face review at any time she wanted it, but indicated that she would need to be the one to initiate it; she did not have to go via her GP. We never heard from her again, and to my knowledge other departments didn't either.

In line with recent NHS initiatives in self-management, General Practitioners are encouraged to help patients to realise their own agency in their lives rather than become increasingly dependent on the traditional pharmacological approach to treatment. Asen et al. (2004) describe simple systemic interventions in their book *Ten Minutes for the Family* that suggest useful ways in which doctors can widen their lenses to consider multiple hypotheses, be more curious about their patients' wider stories and promote self-management in a way that benefits both the patient and the health service. Failure to meet people where they are leads to wasting precious resources as well as exacerbating the health concerns of individuals; we would do well to consider the view that 'Suffering occurs when patients and doctors try to squeeze experience into stories that don't fit. Advice given too quickly deprives people of the opportunity to questions themselves and each other, reflect, and come up with their own answers' (Frank 2013).

I will return to this idea later in this book, but increasingly I have found that actively listening to clients regardless of our professional clinical diagnosis is an important catalyst for change, for self-management and engendering a sense of personal agency: 'In order for families to change one first has to understand and explore the different contexts that the family operates within, otherwise their inability to change is interpreted as resistance, which has been a highly criticised term' (Dell 1982; Keeney 1983; De Shazer 1985).

Systemic theorists demonstrate that 'resistance' in therapy disappears when gentler less power-based therapies are used (Hoffman 1990). This would suggest that resistance can be created by the way therapists present themselves, rather than being an inherent trait of the individual or family. An example in Chapter 5 shows how changing this can alter the dynamic between patient and healthcare worker.

Systemic practice prefers to think about spaces between individuals, and what takes place between them, rather than seeing the problem as only the concern of the individual. In relation to aphasia, this might be seen as aphasia getting in the way of a couple's communication; it is as much the PWA's challenge as the partner's. Such a view promotes likely change in the space between two people, as they are working in a mutually appreciative context (Flaskas et al. 2018).

In Chapter 6, we will see how this focus on the space between the person with aphasia and others can be applied in a very concrete way through Supported Conversation training for families in aphasia therapy. When I started to believe that people generally do the best that they can, given the resources they have, and as I began to be more open to the client's immediate needs and wishes, I found that therapy moved in a more useful direction. Presuming to 'know' and holding fast to diagnostic labels risks wasting resources and missing the person in front of us.

The individual as part of a system

In systemic therapy the concept of the genogram is considered to be key to working with individuals as well as families. Monica McGoldrick has written many books and papers on using family genograms, showing that 'individuals cannot be understood in isolation from one another, but rather as a part of their family, as the family is an emotional unit' (McGoldrick and Gerson 1985). Family therapists typically take a three-generation family tree, created in conjunction with the client to portray not only their core family context but also the dynamics that take place within that family framework. This helps both the client and the therapist to understand the varying influences of diverse aspects of their lives, such as births, deaths, marriages, divorces, beliefs, education, gender, culture, transitions, losses, illness, myths, to name but a few. The genogram helps to identify difficulties and, as McGoldrick suggests, to review expectations, promote acceptable differences, adjust prejudices, and identify family patterns of behaviour. The case study at the end of this chapter will be illustrated with a genogram to show how it helped me to understand and negotiate some of the challenges the client and their family was facing. The genogram is an invaluable tool for use with people with aphasia, given its visual and schematic nature (few words are needed) to help both therapist and client to think about communication within the family, goalsetting, family training, cultural factors and so on.

As part of my work as an SLT, and especially since training in systemic therapy, I have started to attend conferences that are linked to, but not limited to working with adults with aphasia. I have been struck by how many related disciplines discuss useful ideas within the contexts of their own clinical fields, that are highly applicable within aphasia therapy. As mentioned above, the whole premise of systemic understanding is that it considers a variety of sources, instead of the typical linear approach that we tend to see in our continued professional development arenas within health professions. As an SLT who works with adults, for example, I would previously have focussed my continuing professional development (CPD) learning within a narrower academic field. Training as a student of systemic family therapy, I studied alongside a wide range of professions within social care, mental health, eating disorders, nursing, the youth justice system and psychology.

At the National Paediatric Brain Injury Conference 2017, Dr. Jenny Jim, from the Child Brain Injury Rehabilitation Trust spoke about her interest in 'integrating brain and behaviour relationships with a wholistic understanding of a child and young person's context and family'. She practises systemically within the UK's leading charity for children and young people with brain injury and calls for

> A cohesive approach where systemic approaches are incorporated more widely in public health settings can only enhance the experience of patients and their families and may help to address the notions of self-management and efficient use of NHS resources that have been in focus for many years now.

Systemic approaches within services for people with aphasia could transform their experience and the experience of the speech and language therapists who serve them.

Case: Alice

Alice was referred for speech and language therapy 'to improve her word finding and reading ability' following a brain injury. Alice was 65 and had been discharged from a rehabilitation centre with ongoing word finding and reading difficulties. She also had a right-sided hemianopia, was unsteady on her feet due to dizziness and her husband James had recently returned to work. Carers were coming in the morning to help her wash and dress, make breakfast and prepare lunch for her. She and James were living with their 40-year-old son Anthony, who had moved in a year previously whilst saving up his wages to move to his own place in due course. Their daughter Sally was living and working in Bristol. Alice still had frequent hospital appointments on account of her mobility and visual difficulties.

This case illustrates a systemic approach known as narrative therapy and how I applied some aspects of it within speech and language therapy with Alice. Originally developed by Michael White and David Epston (1990), narrative therapy resonated for me with my attempts to work more collaboratively with clients to find a way of living with an impairment. In acquired speech and language disorders, full recovery of function is not always possible.

Social constructionists believe that narratives do not just represent identities, lives and problems, but they actually constitute identities, lives and problems (Carr 1998). When events happen, we make sense of them in the context of our family history, social and cultural contexts, creating meaning from what has happened and living our lives according to that derived meaning (White and Epston 1990).

Systemic and family therapy adopts a 'relational approach' to treating problems in families. By looking at the individual in the context of the family relationships and wider social network, as well as considering the context and actions of the therapist and how they influence one another, positive change can be influenced (Burnham and Harris 1988). When a family member acquires aphasia, or indeed cognitive communication difficulties, this constitutes a 'problem' within the family.

Previously in family therapies, a first-order approach where therapists hold more power and offer treatment to the client prevailed until the mid-1970s, when second-order cybernetics emerged. In speech and language therapy, it could be argued, a 'first-order' approach still tends to characterise therapeutic interventions today.

Narrative therapy focusses on the family system, where a collaborative approach to listening to families in a 'not knowing' way is adopted (Anderson and Goolishian 1992). Alongside our expertise as therapists, this approach allows us to know what we don't know by finding out the client's or family's views and place them as the experts behind the problem they bring to therapy (John Byng-Hall 2005). The narrative approach to therapy considers the presence of power in families as well as the contexts of race, culture, class, gender and sexuality.

The case example below illustrates one way in which a more systemic way of thinking in rehabilitation has been applied; the focus of the work is cognitive-communication difficulty with mild aphasia. Using a genogram helps to position the family as the experts on their situation and to look at the wider context of the family (Hills 2012). The genogram below depicts the family situation as it was when I first met Alice. We can see Alice's current context at a glance, how many professionals were involved, and the nature of the wider family. Genograms might include friends, distant relatives, in fact anything that the person chooses to include.

Speech and language therapy

I visited Alice at home whilst her husband was at work. Alice was petite and immaculately dressed, her home gleaming spotlessly. Nevertheless, she continually apologised for the 'state' of her house. She was engaging, and trying hard to chat, but kept stumbling over words, becoming frustrated and going off on tangents. Informal language assessment indicated mild–moderate aphasia affecting her speech and reading and writing. Alice had reduced insight into apparent attentional and cognitive processing difficulties such as memory, integrating ideas, shifting attention, and understanding longer statements. She used to enjoy word puzzles and word games on her com-

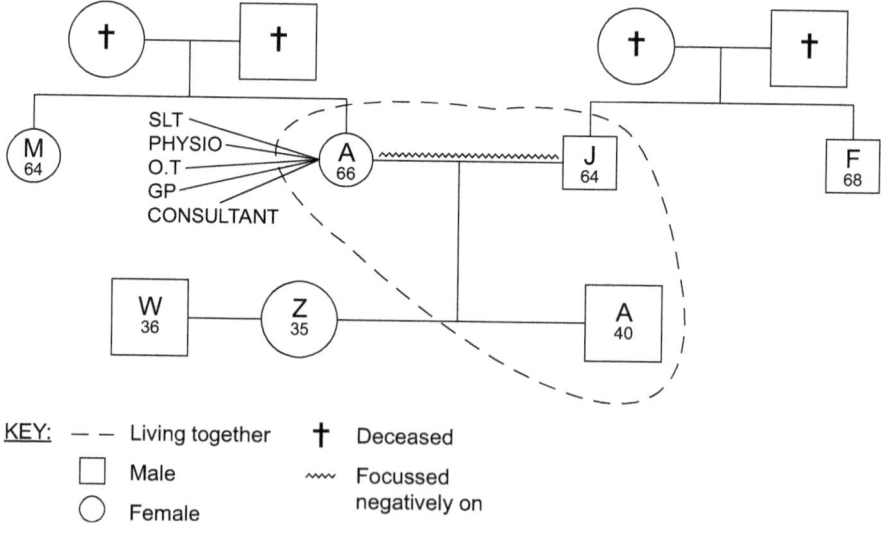

Figure 1.1 A genogram of Alice's family

puter; she also used a smartphone but had lost interest in communicating with friends and acquaintances outside the family. I will not discuss here the wider relationships Alice had with her daughter and her friends; for the purposes of illustration, I will focus on the household only.

We started to focus on Alice's impairments, improving her word-finding skills with word association tasks. She started to progress from reading short passages to the novels she previously enjoyed, but in the form of abridged 'Quick Reads' publications. Gradually, Alice started to keep a diary of events and conversations in order to compensate for short-term memory difficulties. James described to me on the phone the situation as slowly returning to normal, with him working and Sally 'gradually getting better'. Alice and I developed some guidelines for her to offer her family, strategies they could use to help her to feel included in conversations, how to react when she couldn't find her words and so on.

Hardwick (1991) talks about how the referral information may not reflect the reality and the professional network can influence the way the family operates. As Alice's language and reading skills improved, and the professionals and carers involved began to fall away, subtler cognitive difficulties of reduced awareness, insight, tolerance and mood came to the fore. I felt the presence of several professional interventions had been inadvertently 'disguising' some of the cognitive problems until now, when previous routines were resumed, and Alice was receiving fewer interventions.

The presence of son Anthony in the house was not a difficulty prior to the accident, as Alice was able to cope with three-way conversations, but her slower processing skills meant that she misinterpreted information and increasingly friction was occurring in the relationships. James began to describe 'difficulties' in their interactions at the same time as expressing gratitude for her survival and for huge improvements in her language. I subsequently wondered whether he was attempting to find meaning out of the events in terms of God's will, given his strong Christian faith. Alice was frequently getting angry with him and with Anthony, and she had even talked of moving, alone, into her own flat, her expression of which he found very distressing.

Through his GP, James was offered some counselling; his response was that he is the one who offers counselling to others in his church; he does not see himself in the position of receiving counselling. I felt that he did not see that he had a role to play in altering the communicative context at home either; the brain injury belonged to Alice. Reder and Fredman (1996) talk about how we as individuals differ in our relationship to 'help'. James was resistant to seeing himself as someone who needed help, as he was strongly allied to his role as a lay preacher and prayer group leader. He viewed the problem as being Alice's and something to be 'fixed' by the experts.

Brain injury meant a great deal of transition for this family in how they related to one another. I thought about the family's previous internal relationships, which had defined them, or James and Alice as a couple. The family held traditional views as to distribution of labour according to gender within their family. James and Anthony had been taking on some of the 'female' jobs in the house and had needed to support one another during the anxious months when Alice had been critically unwell in hospital.

Minuchin (1974) and Dallos and Procter (1984) refer to power, intimacy and boundaries as the key issues out of which beliefs about how things work are developed over a period of time. With Alice's new way of interacting, such long-held beliefs were being called into question within the family. James and Anthony may have been holding on to the hope that the difficulties would 'resolve' when Alice was 'better'. However, I wanted to encourage them to talk about ways all three of them might start to manage the difficulties now.

In terms of the systemic idea of context of social difference (Burnham 2012), Alice allied herself to me as a woman and mother by talking about how stubborn men are. She complained bitterly that they 'don't bother' to put their cups away. She feels stupid when James and Anthony say something she doesn't fully understand, and she cannot filter out their conversations in the room when trying to watch television. She described how James and Anthony 'talk in front of me but don't make it clear whether I am included or not' so she doesn't know whether to stop and try to listen or not.

When I met Alice, I was aware that she had been a meticulous homemaker in a traditionally female role. Being independent within the house was of great importance to her. For example, she expressed frustration at not being able to hang up the washing as she could not look up without getting very dizzy. I was interested to know about her family and wanted to find shared experience in order to build a rapport or 'collaborative' relationship with her. She wanted to know whether I had children and how I balanced motherhood and work. In thinking about contexts of social difference, I came to appreciate the similarities and differences in our experiences of motherhood and phases of life respectively (her children were adults, and I was a working mother with school-aged children). This necessarily impacted on the ways we talked to each other and how we assumed some shared knowledge. For example, the sense of responsibility in being a parent and some of the frustrations of having to accommodate another person's habits. These entirely 'normal' frustrations had become intolerable for Alice to process following her brain injury.

I began to feel while reading about systemic therapy, however, that the alliance between myself and Alice might become unhelpful to the family as a system. Including James and/or Anthony in the conversations might help to place the difficulties as external to Alice (see below) and to locate those difficulties more between the family members as something everyone has to negotiate or manage. Cecchin (1987) referred to being on nobody's side and on everybody's side in systemic therapy. I chose to reveal that my father was a church minister and I had grown up in a Christian household. I did this to connect with James's strong religious views in some way so that I might bring him into the therapy sessions in order to talk freely about the contexts in which their communication breaks down. I felt he might be interested in a shared experience and see me as someone with whom there was some commonality, however small, hence navigating the relationship to help in some way.

Roberts (2005) advocates transparency where the therapist is 'open about her personal experiences, beliefs, values that may inform therapy'. Self-disclosure is considered to be normalising and reassuring to clients as they see therapists as more real and therefore more open in therapy (Constantine and Kwan 2003).

In further joint sessions with James and Alice, we talked about their experience of the communication difficulties. I used circular questioning (Penn 1982) to find out about whose difficulty this is they are struggling with; asking questions which depend on a response in order to formulate further questions, to change the person's perspective on their situation and stimulate new thinking about the problem (Dallos and Draper 2010). I asked Alice what she thought was different in James's day-to-day life since the accident compared to previously. Her response was surprising to both me and James, as we heard that she could not see that his life had in any way been altered, only that he was not talking properly to her or explaining things clearly, treating her like a child. James was able then to talk about how worried he was about her when she was in hospital, while he was at work and when she was recovering at home, as well as his sadness about her memory difficulties making it hard for them to talk about past experiences together or even recognise places they had visited in their youth.

All the family were grieving from their own position. James and Alice had been approaching the consequences of the brain injury from very different places. The rules on which their lives operated previously were now bringing them into conflict as their conversations took place from different viewpoints. Alice was not able to see things from James's viewpoint due to her rigid thinking process, but James assumed the problem was 'her' brain injury and she needed restoring through therapy, rather than him changing his interaction style to accommodate the changes in Alice's communication behaviour. Both Alice and James identified themselves as being competent and yet things broke down frequently. For some time, they had waited for things to be restored, (as reinforced by health professionals caring for Alice?) but now, it was the communication styles that needed to change.

Externalising the problem in the narrative tradition involves helping the clients to see themselves as separate from the problem (Carr 1998). Alice and James decided that the thing between them was called 'misunderstand-ing'. Alice said James didn't explain himself properly and James said he often felt misunderstood. My intention in externalising the communica-tion difficulty was so that James and Alice might start to see themselves as jointly trying to manage the difficulty which does not just lie with Alice. (She is often oblivious to the effects of the cognitive impairment.) As we talked about misunderstanding, which came between them now and again, James described it as doing a jigsaw puzzle; the main items in the picture are easier to find and piece together but then, suddenly, you try to do the sky and it is hard to make the pieces fit. He used this analogy to explain that often communication goes well and then seemingly out of the blue Alice doesn't understand, and he is reminded of the brain injury and the loss of Alice-as-she-was. Alice was able to relate to this image and became more concerned about how James was feeling about her and began to see he was trying to connect with her, rather than deliberately 'being awkward'.

Asking 'relative influence questions' in order to find a unique outcome helped me to identify, for example, the instances where Alice finds it hard to understand James and those where she finds it easy to understand him, when James and Anthony talking together is distracting and when it isn't.

I asked both about what they wanted for each other in future. They both identified more self-confidence for Alice, especially in participating in their church group. We talked about sharing something about misunderstanding and being misunderstood with the group and sharing Alice's fear of saying the wrong words. They both thought they might seek support from others, and hope for reassurance that friends want to hear from Alice.

A key practice in narrative therapy of linking the new story to the past and extending into the future (White and Epston 1990) was useful in working with Alice and James. I asked some excavating (recalling forgotten experience) questions such as 'If I had met you 5 years ago how would you be talking about where you will go for your holiday compared to how you do that now?' Then, 'Given what you have talked about in terms of giving each other time to talk and writing key things down as you do so, how do you think you will be talking about where your next holiday will be?'

Reflexive questions such as 'What does this say about how you will plan things together in future?' were aimed at influencing James and Alice to reorganise their view of 'misunderstanding' in a different way so they can communicate effectively, whilst retaining their enjoyment of holidays and indeed other ordinary life events. Alice volunteered that she would keep a diary on holiday so that they could reminisce at a later date in case she had forgotten things. Such ideas were opening up communication with James rather than shutting it down as previously. James had some strategies with which to reengage with his wife differently.

After our sessions, I summarised our discussions in writing to James and Alice separately ('using literary means', White and Epston 1990); I offered the idea of keeping the jigsaw idea in mind as a way of 'doing the sky pieces together' in the future.

Through working with this family, who had acquired a communication disorder, I started to position myself and the client within a more collaborative stance. It enabled me to develop similar perspectives with other clients and I started to observe people coming up with far better solutions than I could have dreamt of for them. Was this speech and language therapy or was it counselling, or was it both or neither?

The narrative approach described here, of listening for dominant stories, trying to map how the problem influences people's lives and how it affects their relationships and how people inadvertently maintain the problem (White and Epston 1990), sits comfortably with my own personal and professional context. I thought about the invisible nature of Alice's injury and how we had worked to make it more visible and voiced through this process. The key change for Alice, myself and the family in this case was bringing James into the sessions. Now they both view the problem as there for the long-term, but shared; separate from who they are, and a part of their past as well as their future together.

References

Anderson, H. and Goolishian, H. (1988) Human systems as linguistic systems: Preliminary and evolving ideas about the implications for clinical theory. *Family Process*. Dec;27(4): 371–393.

Anderson, H. and Goolishian, H. (1992) 'The client is the expert: A not-knowing approach to therapy'. In S. McNamee and K. J. Gergen (Eds), *Therapy as Social Construction* (pp. 25–39). Sage.

Asen, E., Tomson, D., Young, V. and Tomson, P. (2004) *Ten Minutes for the Family: Systemic Interventions in Primary Care*. Routledge.

Bateson, G. (1972) *Steps to an Ecology of Mind: Mind and Nature*. Ballantine Books.

Benedetti, F. (2008) *Placebo Effects: Understanding the Mechanisms in Health and Disease*. Oxford University Press.

Biletzki, A. and Matar, A. (2020) 'Ludwig Wittgenstein', *The Stanford Encyclopaedia of Philosophy* (Spring 2020 Edition), Edward N. Zalta (Ed.)

Burnham, J. (2012) 'Developments in social GRRRAAACCEEESSS'. In I-B Krause (Ed.), *Culture and Reflexivity in Systemic Psychotherapy: Mutual Perspectives*. Karnac.

Burnham, J. and Harris, Q. (1988) 'Systemic family therapy: The Milan approach'. In E. Street and W. Dryden (Eds), *Family Therapy in Britain*. Open University Press.

Byng-Hall, J. (2005) Attachment and human survival. *Journal of Family Therapy*, 27(1): 97–98.

Capra, F. (2018) Homage to Gregory Bateson. Available at https://batesoninstitute.org/gregory-bateson/

Capra, F. and Luisi, P. L. (2014) *The Systems View of Life. A Unifying Vision*. Cambridge University Press.

Carr, A. (1998) Michael White's narrative therapy. *Contemporary Family Therapy*, 20, 485–503

Cecchin, G. (1987) Hypothesising, circularity and neutrality revisited: An invitation to curiosity, *Family Process*, 26 (4): 405–414.

Constantine, M. G. and Kwan, K. L. K. (2003) Cross-cultural considerations of therapist self-disclosure. *Journal of Clinical Psychology*, 59(5): 581–588.

Dallos, R. and Draper, R. (2010) *An Introduction to Family Therapy. Systemic Theory and Practice*. Third edition. McGraw-Hill Education.

Dallos, R. and Procter, H. G. (1984) Family processes: An interactional view. *Social Psychology: Creating a Social World Block 1: Development, Experience and Behaviour in a Social World*. Open University Press.

Dell, P. E. (1982) Beyond homeostasis: Toward a concept of coherence, *Family Process*, 21: 21–42.

De Shazer, S. (1985) *Keys to Solution in Brief Therapy*. W. W. Norton.

Flaskas, C., Mason, B. and Perlesz, A. (Eds) (2018) *The Space Between: Experience, Context, and Process in the Therapeutic Relationship*. Routledge.

Frank, A. W. (2013) *The Wounded Storyteller: Body, Illness, and Ethics*. Second edition. University of Chicago Press.

Gurman, A. S. and Kniskern, D. P. (1978) Deterioration in marital and family therapy: Empirical, clinical, and conceptual issues. *Family Process*, 17: 3–20.

Hardwick, P. J. (1991) Families and the professional network: An attempted classification of professional network actions which can hinder change. *Journal of Family Therapy*, 13(2): 187–205.

Harrington, A. (2008). *The Cure Within: A History of Mind-Body Medicine*. W. W. Norton.

Hills, J. (2012) *Introduction to Systemic and Family Therapy*. Macmillan International Higher Education.

Hoffman, L. (1990) Constructing realities: An art of lenses. *Family Process*, 29: 1–12.

Keeney, B. (1983) *Aesthetics of Change*. Basic Books.

Mason, B. (1993) Towards positions of safe uncertainty. *Human Systems: The Journal of Systemic Consultation and Management*, 4: 189–200.

McGoldrick, M. and Gerson, R. (1985) *Genograms in Family Assessment*. W. W. Norton.

Milz, H. (2014) 'Integrative practice in healthcare and healing'. In F. Capra and P. L. Luisi (Eds), *A Systems View of Life. A Unifying Vision*. Cambridge University Press.

Minuchin, S. (1974) *Families and Family Therapy*. Harvard University Press.

Parsons, T. (1985) *Talcott Parsons on Institutions and Social Evolution: Selected Writings*. University of Chicago Press.

Penn, P. (1982) Circular questioning. *Family Process*, 21(3): 267–280.

Ramig, L. O., Halpern, A., Spielman, J., Fox, C. and Freeman, K. (2018). Speech treatment in Parkinson's disease: Randomized controlled trial (RCT). *Movement Disorders*, 33(11): 1777–1791.

Reder, P. and Fredman, G. (1996) The relationship to help: Interacting beliefs about the treatment process. *Clinical Child Psychology and Psychiatry*, 1(3): 457–467.

Roberts, J. (2005) Transparency and self-disclosure in family therapy: Dangers and possibilities. *Family Process*, Mar;44(1): 45–63.

White, M. and Epston, D. (1990) *Narrative Means to Therapeutic Ends*. W. W. Norton.

2

A brief overview of aphasia therapy

This chapter will briefly summarise the development of some of the approaches to aphasia therapy over the last 30 years as well as the current nature and availability of aphasia services in this country.

The case study which follows will be an example of my work with a woman with aphasia in a more traditional, or 'non-systemic' way, prior to training in systemic therapy. I hope that I now work in a more informed and useful manner than I did then! By contrasting this (flawed) case with the systemic approaches adopted in later case studies, I hope readers will start to appreciate the benefits to be gained in this field.

Traditionally, speech and language therapists (SLTs) are considered to be skilled in the therapeutic treatment of aphasia. Aphasia is caused by an injury to the brain. A stroke, either where there is a blockage of blood flow to the brain, or a small bleed in the brain can cause aphasia, depending on the location of the stroke in the brain. Following a stroke, the language processing systems are permanently interrupted, to some extent in nearly all cases. However, recovery does occur in varying degrees in different individuals. A CT scan following a stroke usually identifies areas of damage and can loosely predict the nature of aphasia likely to present itself. Traumatic brain injury can also result in aphasia and because such injuries are less focal, the aphasia may be accompanied by wider cognitive processing challenges, such as memory, attention, and dysexecutive function.

Aphasia is not an articulatory disorder, in spite of the impression that the person with aphasia is struggling to form sounds and words in speech. There is no communication aid that can replace the incredibly complex, rich language system most of us are fortunate enough to be born with.

DOI: 10.4324/9781003178613-2

The philosopher Philip Wheelwright (1968) once said, 'if reality is largely fluid and half-paradoxical, then steel nets are not the best thing for taking samples of it'. I believe this to be true of the fluid and paradoxical nature of language and thought. Communication aids that depict multiple images and words which are handed out to people with aphasia are usually done in order to satisfy the needs of the nurse or therapist in having delivered a 'tool' (however ineffectual) and it buys in to the 'fix it' model of medical care, that colleagues and families expect.

To work with aphasia demands, at the very least, an understanding of clinical linguistics, neurology and an element of psychology. This is because aphasia is highly variable to individuals, as are the ways in which people respond to the onset of such a devastating event. Over 27 years, I have not seen two people with aphasia who are alike and so it comes as no surprise that research has focussed on single case study design. However, at the point of delivery, health services often offer a 'one size fits all' approach which often fails to meet the needs of clients, and, I would argue, of this client group in particular.

Brady et al. (2016) demonstrated in their systemic review that 'each individual case demonstrated a unique type and degree of emotional or psychosocial response to stroke and aphasia'. As a result, 'rehabilitation progress, psychosocial and emotional adjustment could not be anticipated or assumed. This suggests that each individual should be considered unique, patterns of recovery being dependent on impairment, disability and handicap across neural, cognitive, behavioural, psychosocial and cognitive domains.' They concluded that the idiosyncratic nature of all these factors confirms the value of single case studies in aphasia research.

Furthermore, they demonstrated evidence of the effectiveness of speech and language therapy (SLT) for people with aphasia (PWA) following stroke in terms of improved functional communication, reading, writing, and expressive language compared with no therapy. The reality, however, is that availability and quality of aphasia therapy is also highly variable. In addition, I think that we do not sufficiently consider the holistic improvement and adjustment following aphasia that is made many years after the brain injury; the focus is too short-term, and therefore inadequate.

Diagnosis

Diagnostic categories of aphasia are available that have traditionally been used in teaching (e.g., Broca's, Wernicke's, conduction, global, transcortical) and some clinicians hold to these descriptors very firmly. I am not one of them. The labels refer to either the area of damage in the brain, the configuration of errors the person makes, or infer that the person has damage in every area of language processing (global aphasia).

The difficulty with diagnostic labels from a systemic point of view, is that they encourage one to fit the patient to the label and ignore aspects of the person that do not fit tidily into that description. Furthermore, the labels refer to a particular point in time only.

For example, a Wernicke's type aphasia can be described as largely fluent and possibly jargonistic, whereas Broca's aphasia is normally non-fluent, with greater awareness and more struggle to find and produce words. In reality, I have seen patients who present with the former type of aphasia and develop non-fluency as they progress over time. I have worked with 'global aphasia', where there is clear progress in language processing and excellent development of paralinguistic and nonverbal communication in social contexts. Are these terms really meaningful still?

I encourage students to explore and merely describe the presentation of the aphasia as it appears in the person they are treating. If they recognise that what they observe fits that particular time, and that particular situation and may alter in different context, they are likely to better understand aphasia. Readiness to observe, actively listen and change one's mind is essential when working with aphasia if one is to get a true understanding of the nature of the condition.

Aphasia therapy sits firmly within the professional role of the speech and language therapist who works with adults in clinical settings, either in hospitals, rehabilitation units or in the community. Associated, as it often is, with brain injuries, patients may have additional swallowing difficulties (dysphagia). The last 30 years has seen SLTs become increasingly involved clinically in assessing and treating these patients, to the extent that the more urgent need for feeding safely has prioritised these cases over those with aphasia.

Along with this development, in my view, is that increased training in dysphagia management, and LSVT (see Chapter 1), has given therapists a greater sense of certainty and competency, in that such difficulties can be managed in short interventions and with specific, measurable goals.

Historical background to aphasia

In the mid-nineteenth century the French surgeon Paul Broca started to link damage to the physical brain with intellectual, cognitive and psychological functions. The frontal part of the left hemisphere of the brain was identified by Paul Broca in 1861 as controlling speech function. It was understood that location was important to function, but only for diagnosis at this stage, rather than remediation. By 1948 Kurt Goldstein was writing about aphasic syndromes and possible therapeutic approaches for relearning language (Goldstein 1948). The following 50 years saw a number of emerging therapies.

Key approaches in the treatment of aphasia that are still in use today are outlined below. Many of these can be and are used interchangeably, although it has been my observation over the last 20 years that graduate therapists will tend to favour one approach over another: often according to either their training institution's preferences or that of their first work setting.

Speech and language therapy students are less likely to have had training in the psycholinguistic approach to aphasia therapy, or if they have, are less likely to feel confident in applying it in the clinical context now compared with 20 years ago. Graduates and placement students report lack of confidence in working with people with aphasia and will often choose to focus on the other areas of the profession where more objective or 'script' based approaches to remediation can be adopted.

Functional communication

In the 1970s, Audrey Holland began to focus on 'functional communication' rather than 'linguistic accuracy' for individuals with aphasia. She was aware that PWA could often 'communicate' better than they could 'talk' (Holland 1979; Armstrong and Ferguson 2010). This approach encouraged people to explore everyday ways of communicating for people with aphasia, such as using gestures to convey meaning, instead of just testing people on their ability to do language tasks at a desk.

Psycholinguistics

In the 1980s, cognitive neuropsychology-based therapy came to the fore with a more detailed description of the development of aphasiology from neurolinguistics (Caplan 1987; Jones 1986). This is still part of some practice, today, and forms the basis of the excellent therapy workstation, Cuespeak (Cuespeak Ltd). Psycholinguistic therapy allowed an analysis of precise areas of linguistic breakdown and targeted interventions supported by research largely into single case studies. Some assessment tools such as the Psycholinguistic Assessment of Language Processing in Aphasia (Kay et al. 1992) started to offer the therapist a way of thinking about separate areas of linguistic breakdown and devising tasks that tapped into these areas.

I was fortunate enough to have been trained under the tutelage of the esteemed Eirian Jones (1986) whose own highly analytical linguistic approach did not neglect the social and family experience of the person with aphasia, contrary to the beliefs of many proponents of the social disability model which soon followed. Eirian Jones's work focussed on hypothesis formation in language assessment: word finding difficulties were described

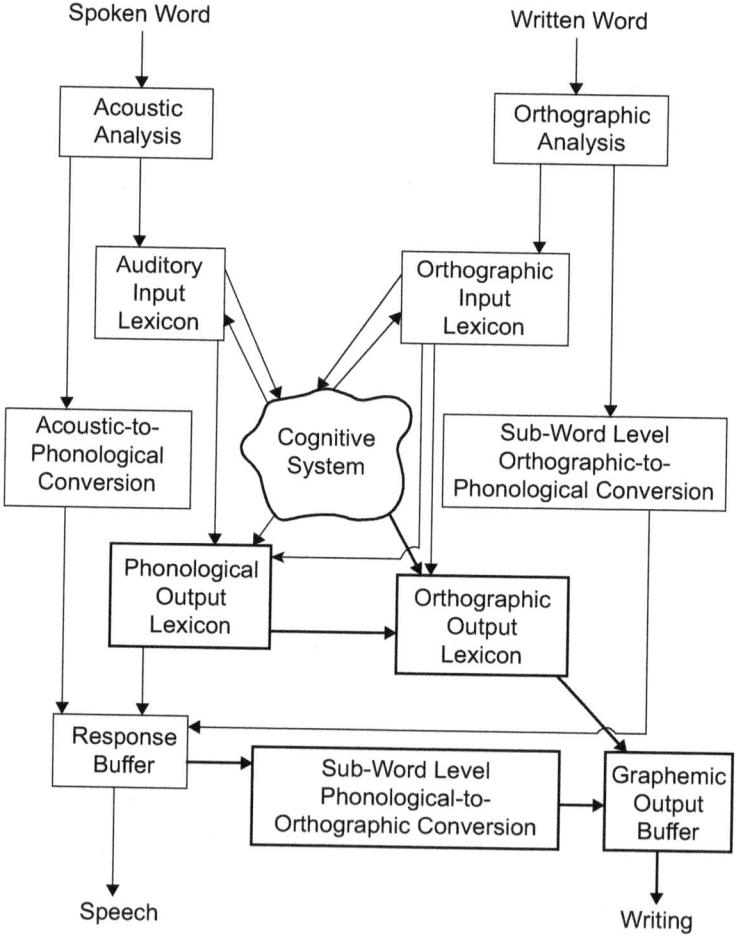

Figure 2.1 Cognitive-linguistic model of single word processing
Source: Patterson and Shewell (1987)

with reference to a neuropsychological model of single word processing (Fig.2.1) based on patterns of errors (1986).

This model, as well as the updated version of this model, guided therapists to think about different areas of breakdown, such as the following:

Semantic deficit (impaired spoken and written word production and impaired comprehension)

Phonological output lexicon (impaired spoken/intact written naming, spoken and reading comprehension

Phonological assembly (all spoken production tasks affected)

Articulatory planning (impairment to all spoken production tasks)

Whitworth et al. (2005) clearly stated that a neuropsycholinguistic approach to therapy should be only part of the holistic framework for working with aphasia and used within a total communication framework. In spite of this, there seems to have been little meeting of minds; narrative in clinics and on courses has tended to be dichotomous, as if one approach excludes the other.

Social disability model

In the 1990s the social model philosophy of disability emerged. This considered the identity of the PWA in the context of their social environment (Pound et al. 2000; Simmons-Mackie and Damico 1996). To develop a socially broader, more ecologically valid perspective, they exhorted aphasiologists to view the behaviours of individuals with aphasia from a socially sensitive perspective. Environmental factors could influence communication behaviours positively or negatively, and this was considered a better focus than judging behaviour based on preconceived notions of 'appropriateness' or otherwise.

Such social model approaches took a philosophical stance which claimed to challenge power relationships between service providers and people with disabilities by addressing social exclusion and isolation, valuing the lived experience and expertise of disabled people, collaborative practice, authentic involvement of the person with aphasia in the decision-making process and working on practical, worthwhile experiences in the clinic (Pound et al. 2000).

In 2001 an international standard to describe and measure health and disability was created by the World Health Organisation and endorsed by

191 member states: the International Classification of Functioning, Disability & Health (ICF). The ICF conceptualises a person's level of functioning as a dynamic interaction between her or his health conditions, environmental factors, and personal factors. It is a biopsychosocial model of disability, based on an integration of the social and medical models of disability which aims to address and consider the relationships between the following:

- the body functions and structures of people and impairments thereof (functioning at the level of the body);
- the activities of people (functioning at the level of the individual) and the activity limitations they experience;
- the participation or involvement of people in all areas of life, and the participation restrictions they experience (functioning of a person as a member of society); and
- the environmental factors which affect these experiences (and whether these factors are facilitators or barriers).

Translated into an approach for aphasia therapy, therapists might target speech work, improved conversational ability at home, group role play work, lack of communication partners at home.

National guidelines that aphasia therapists follow include the Royal College of Physicians *National Clinical Guideline for Stroke* (2008), which states that the aims of rehabilitation are to 'facilitate adaptation to disability, to promote social and community integration, and to maximize well-being and quality of life'.

The National Stroke Strategy (2007) states 'The aim is to achieve a good quality of life for individuals, their carers and relatives, and to support independent living', while the National Service Framework for Older People (2001) promotes person-centred care with the ideal that 'NHS and social care services treat older people as individuals and enable them to make choices about their own care.'

'The Life Participation Approach to Aphasia'

'The Life Participation Approach to Aphasia' (LPAA: Chapey et al. 2000) is a general philosophy and model of service delivery, that 'supports individuals with aphasia and others affected by it in achieving their immediate and longer-term life goals'. From initial assessment in hospital to the point at which the PWA no longer chooses to have therapy, it emphasises re-engagement in life and tries to empower the PWA to collaborate on their therapeutic treatments, with the aim of returning to an active life.

Therapists soon began to look more closely at the important role of training conversation partners with skills to support people with aphasia.

Supported Conversation for Adults with Aphasia was developed by the Aphasia Institute in Canada. University College London also has Better Conversations (Beeke et al. 2015), an online training tool for professionals or individuals to learn how best to communicate with and support someone who has aphasia to communicate with others. Its goal is to improve interactive experiences for people who have trouble speaking or understanding language, the focus being on the communication partner, and the immediate environment, not the person with aphasia. Such training asks the person with aphasia and the communication partner to work together to improve communication, acknowledging that conversation is an important part of life participation. It assumes that the person with aphasia is competent or knows more than they can say and trains the communication partner to help the person with aphasia to get and give information.

Supported conversation uses total communication. This means that communication by any means is encouraged, not just speaking. Drawing writing, gesturing, and facial expression are all valid. Conversation partners are asked to use a normal volume of voice, write down key words, wait and listen, use drawing, summarise their understanding, use closed questions, and so on as means by which to ensure more successful interactions. Similar approaches such as Conversational Coaching for Aphasia and Supported Communication Intervention are offered in America.

Whilst the aims of these models are admirable and ones I fully endorse, I will argue that without the necessary skills that systemic training provides, they do not deliver what they set out to achieve. Some families struggle to make the adjustment to using supported conversation techniques and their reasons for this are many and varied. When this happens families and therapists feel frustrated, and clients can be left experiencing a sense of failure. My premise is, that without a therapist who is skilled in aphasia therapy as well as in family systems, interventions often merely act as sticking plaster until the therapy has come to an end.

Enderby has worked tirelessly for many years to improve the evidence base of aphasia therapy but, alongside that, has always argued for the ongoing recognition of the role of expertise (Enderby 2004), a view which I wholeheartedly endorse.

As Sackett et al. (1996) note, 'Without clinical expertise, practice risks becoming tyrannized by evidence, for even excellent external evidence may be inapplicable to or inappropriate for an individual patient.'

Neural plasticity

Both impairment and non-impairment approaches to aphasia therapy are based partly on the principles of a 'use it or lose it' and 'Use it and improve it' approach to neural plasticity (Kleim and Jones 2008). Inadequate use of a brain system is thought to lead to further degradation of function; how much of this is due to the emotional and psychological effects of non-use cannot be proven, however. We believe that using a specific function will enhance it. We know that behavioural experience can enhance per-formance, and probably through brain plasticity, but that there are certain things that help. For example, Kleim and Jones outline the following prin-ciples of brain plasticity which we might consider in the brain that has received an injury:

Specificity – the type of the trained task influences the nature of neural plas-ticity and behavioural changes are dependent upon specific kinds of experience

Repetition – learning a skill and practising that skill again and again over time is helpful

Intensity – training intensity can influence neural plasticity

Time – there may be time windows in which therapy is particularly effective in directing reactive plasticity, however we do not know enough about when these might be in different individuals

Salience – behaviours are more like to be remembered if they are emotion-ally or psychologically salient, and these will also influence motivation and engagement

Age – neuroplastic responses are altered in the aged brain.

Transference – training in one area can affect plasticity in other areas of behaviour

Interference – plasticity in response to one area can interfere with learning in another area

(Kleim and Jones 2008)

Errorless learning

An errorless learning approach to therapy in aphasia has been favoured in recent years. Hebbian-based learning maintains that neurons that 'fire together are wired together', meaning that their connections are made stronger. For this reason, therapists may want to avoid reinforcing errors, for example in naming items, an errorless approach might involve a client being shown a picture, seeing the written name and hearing the name of it spoken aloud. They might be asked to repeat the word several times and given the word and sound in order to aid their chances of a correct response.

Ylvisaker et al. (2006) thought that this approach was beneficial for clients who make lots of errors and have additional memory difficulties, or for whom confidence building was of particular importance. Indeed, clients often prefer this approach, which in my view brings up some of the ideas under discussion throughout this book about power based therapeutic relationships. Studies seem to suggest that, objectively, both approaches are equally effective at improving word finding (Conroy et al. 2009).

Intensive therapy

There is some indication from systematic reviews of clinical research that therapy at high intensity, high dose or over a longer period may be beneficial (Brady et al. 2016). ILAT (Intensive Language Action Therapy) is one that has demonstrated efficacy of intensive therapy for chronic post-stroke aphasia.

ILAT is based upon the theoretical linguistic premise that the primary function of language emerges from its everyday use (Tomasello et al. 2005; Wittgenstein 1956). The intensive training constitutes up to 30 hours of practice in under two weeks and is focussed on the training of language skills in the context of communication and social interaction (Difrancesco et al. 2012). Studies by Egorova et al. (2013, 2014, 2016) showed that asking for an object elicits stronger neurological signals in the language and motor regions of the brain than just naming the items. Interest in this approach was strengthened by evidence for the short- and long-term benefits, even when delivered years following the onset of the disease (Meinzer et al. 2005; Pulvermüller et al. 2001). In practice, high-intensity and high dose interventions may not be acceptable to all; they demand extensive resources from service delivery as well as access by the patient to centres. The aphasia therapy workstation Cuespeak, however, provides a theoretically sound means of providing intensive therapy at home with support of a therapist and goes a considerable way to enabling higher doses of contextually relevant therapy to be accessed.

Many additional language therapies may form part of the therapist's toolbox, but will not be described in detail here, including Gestural Facilitation of Naming, PACE therapy, Semantic feature Analysis treatment and Verb network strengthening treatment (VNest). Group therapies are offered in some places, varying from two to many participants, although the nature and content of such groups varies widely.

In many countries around the world services for people with aphasia either do not exist or are extremely sparse. Aphasia United is an international organisation established in 2011 that seeks to create partnerships and shared understanding about aphasia between researchers, clinicians and people with aphasia. They created 'Best Practice Recommendations' which are backed by evidence of varying degrees (see the list of 'Primary Sources' on their website, available at www.aphasiaunited.org/wp-content/uploads/2016/05/English-Aphasia-United-Best-Practices-Recommendations1.pdf). These will be examined further in Chapter 8. Below is a summary of their premise for aphasia therapy intervention.

> People with aphasia have preserved pre-onset intelligence, but intelligence can be masked by difficulty communicating. It should never be assumed that a person with aphasia is mentally incompetent. People with aphasia are typically able to make decisions and participate in activities if information or activities are made communicatively accessible. People with aphasia and their family members have the right to relevant services designed for the individual to enhance communication and participation in life activities of choice. Health care services for people with aphasia should be person-cantered and collaborative.

At the time of writing, the Royal College of Speech and Language Therapists does not hold any data that shows the percentage of qualified SLT's working with aphasia, compared with the numbers who work with dysphagia, or indeed other conditions associated with an adult caseload of patients. There does not appear to be data either, that shows whether there is a reduction in the number of therapists who specialise in the treatment of aphasia. My working experience alone suggests that it is quite significant, although aphasia researchers seem to be numerous.

Aphasia is a fascinating condition, and students are often drawn to speech and language therapy because they want to be able to remediate difficulties; however, when faced with the complexity of aphasia, I believe they feel helpless and lose interest, in favour of other clinical treatments.

My experience is that provision varies widely in terms of availability of aphasia therapy, time post-injury at which therapy is offered, level of skill offered by the therapist, types of therapy offered, intensity of therapy offered, the philosophy and personal beliefs of the therapist, clinical training background, level of support from managers of services and so on. There are no doubt centres that offer excellent therapy and support. PWA who live in university towns may have access to therapy provided as part of research programmes; however they are few and far between. Interestingly, some research studies, such as ILAT referred to above, compared their forms of treatment with 'traditional therapy'. I often wonder what constitutes 'traditional therapy', given that visiting a range of clinics in this country alone will offer up highly varied experiences of this notion!

Centres such as the Aphasia Institute in Canada and Connect (formerly in London and sadly no longer) have been successful, precisely because they focus on aphasia only, rather than picking up clients with aphasia when they get to the bottom of their list of more 'urgent' neurological patients. I will be raising the question in this book, of whether aphasia therapists should be just that; whether a specific set of skills are required for this role in order for it to be meaningful as well cost-effective.

The 'ivory tower' of the acute hospital setting in the UK means that acute medicine is prioritised, and that aphasia therapy, whilst important, fails to give the client an idea of the 'whole story', for their work does not usually extend beyond the inpatient stay, or if it does, it is usually in very limited outpatient sessions. Work carried out by SLTs in this setting, whilst it might be excellent, does not often focus on the longer-term picture, as it is often not within the specialist experience of the clinician.

Whilst aphasia receives some form of intervention through ESD (early supported discharge), I struggle to see what can be achieved in six weeks by rehabilitation assistants for what may be a lifelong condition with massive adjustment processes to be worked through. The patient leaves hospital with the assurance, in some areas, of six weeks of 'early supported discharge'. This is a time during which the PWA and their family have burning questions about prognosis, about the intricate complexities of language processing and we expect a generic rehabilitation worker to be able to offer suitable answers to such questions? At this point the patient doesn't know that it might be all they get, and that they will not necessarily have recovered after this time period. Further, they do not always know that this will not be delivered by an aphasia therapist, but by a generic rehabilitation assistant who doesn't know the answers to the questions 'Am I doing ok?', 'When will I get my speech back?', 'Am I going to read again?'. Some will say they don't know, others will generously attempt an optimistic answer, such as 'Of course, just keep trying hard you will be fine'.

The nuances of the therapeutic relationship, feedback, understanding of the processes involved in language are absent for the assistant who is placed in the position of supporting the person who has lost the very thing that makes them human, and represents their identity: language. The assistant can't be held responsible for lack of progress in those extraordinarily specific six weeks, so the responsibility is felt by the patient; the person who is struggling to hold on to their sense of self, communicate their fears to their friends and family, ask questions, express feelings, and so on. Again, applying a sticking plaster to a serious wound is unlikely to be effective in the longer term.

Having received ESD, patients often have to wait considerable lengths of time to reach the top of the community services waiting list, unless a proactive approach to the management of aphasia is taken. By the time they reach the clinic, they are already anxious, relationships may have broken down and they express beliefs or 'truths' about aphasia recovery that fly in the face of the evidence. A common example of this is 'If I'm not better in 6 months I never will be', which was told to a client of mine by a stroke doctor at the time of writing this book.

The community therapist, who will eventually receive the client, and already faced with clients with a wide range of swallowing and communication disorders of varying aetiology, is frankly often left struggling to see the tip of the iceberg.

Many community services are focussed on goal setting and will limit therapy sessions, either to a finite number, or to achievement of a specified goal. I will be talking about my reservations about this approach, based on my own experiences, in Chapter 6.

I would argue that the dichotomy of impairment versus functional therapy aphasia is artificial and no longer helpful; the speech and language therapist needs to be cognisant of the linguistic system, the family system, and their own therapist-client system. An understanding of the range of resources for working with aphasia, brought together by a systemic approach would ensure a flexible, truly client-centred service for people with aphasia and their families.

Case: Babs

Babs was 58 when she had a left-sided stroke in 2007, leaving her with severe aphasia and right-sided weakness. A mother to two adult children, and married to Harry for many years, Babs loved her work in a day centre for the elderly community, organising the centre and running activities there. She was a talented artist, enjoying watercolour painting and calligraphy. Harry was already happily retired and spent hours in his workshop, on his computer and listening to music.

My intervention with this couple is hard to describe; I feel disappointed that I failed to offer the insights and understanding that I would offer today. Nonetheless, its inclusion serves to illustrate progression to a more systemic approach in later case studies described in this book.

Following her stroke, Babs had received six weeks of outpatient speech and language therapy before being discharged. She felt frustrated that she was not making faster progress. She and Harry reported that many friends had fallen away when Babs returned home, and they both felt devasted when people they knew well avoided them in the street. A new start in a new town and nearer to Bab's sister seemed a good idea. Babs and Harry relocated.

Babs walked unsteadily into the room, supported by Harry. They thanked me for agreeing to see them despite having had speech therapy previously elsewhere. Harry waited for Babs to talk which she struggled to do, and she immediately became frustrated and tearful. I explained that I would work with them on her aphasia, that I realised her ability to think, and they looked hopeful. Comparing my image of how Harry had described Babs before her stroke to the unhappy, frustrated but nevertheless warm-hearted lady before me, and, given their story of feeling let down I desperately wanted to be of help. I summoned up my best aphasiology skills, carried out some selected language assessments and embarked on a twice weekly programme of therapy over a period of four months.

Pre-therapy assessments 30/10/07

Palpa 2.5 Word Repetition 40/40
Palpa 2.8 Reading aloud 20/20
Palpa 3.1 Sentence Comprehension 26/30 repetitions required 50% of the time
Core meanings of verbs ok, errors = reversible directional active verbs suggesting mapping difficulty.
Written verb naming 16/20
Palpa 53 Spoken picture naming 38/40

> *Cinderella was . . . lived in a house with a stepmother and her... daughters she has a lot of chores to the . . . house um . . . they (laugh) the ball has invited her step step sister she had a lot of work in the (gestured sleeves – clothing? In the house?) clothes (ballgowns?) yes! Ballgowns she had to sew them up and hair their . . . (do their hair?) yes, yes and she felt very sad when um he the stepsisters went had to go to the ball then she'd worked very sad she wasn't sad a poor attire*

Verbs (6) live, have, invited, sew, feel, go
Nouns (12) Cinderella, house, stepmother, daughters, chores, stepsister, work, hair, attire

Therapy programme

Babs was very frustrated by her word finding and sentence planning difficulties. She wanted to understand where it was going wrong and what she could do about it. I believe that a psycholinguistic framework helps people with aphasia to understand that it is not their fault that attempts at communication keep failing and that there are real processes, about which we understand only a little, admittedly, that can improve through therapy and also be compensated for in real-life personal interactions.

If the whole effect of aphasia on a person and their family is an overwhelming mystery (which is how it is frequently reported), how can people begin to understand why and how compensatory strategies will work, and more importantly, know which ones will not work before they try hard to implement them and then feel shame and disappointment when they don't work?

My personal view is that we should share our knowledge with our clients as far as we can and work together to restore and compensate simultaneously. If family members are present for some of this therapy, they too will start to see the competence of their loved one and their many areas of strength,

- Mapping therapy: subject-verb-object sentences, identifying verbs and thematic roles of nouns, creating sentences from verbs,
- Constraint induced action therapy (based on ILAT) – high frequency nouns e.g., doctor, church, post office, coffee, cat, family names, three groups of verbs transitive (1 argument), two arguments etc.
- Sentence planning tasks, particularly with directional, 2-argument verbs, e.g., learn, instruct, teach, chase. Discussed perspectives using diagrams and it took a long time for Babs to identify 'who was doing to whom'.
- Higher level semantic work to boost verb semantic retrieval: verbs of movement, possession and location in particular.
- Semantic circles, odd one out (semantically related distractors) Babs tended to retrieve nouns in place of the verb in conversations, and this seemed to interrupt her attempts to find the correct verb.
- Synonyms
- Formulating Wh- questions
- Using famous paintings for giving a title of the painting and describing the main event in the picture.
- Procedural tasks, devising instructions for painting with a sheet of nouns to use

I must stress that during this therapy period, attention was indeed given to how Babs was feeling, and how her participation in life was affected by her disability.

I often used to create my own model of a pie chart (influenced by Kagan's Life Participation Approach) which we would populate with all the activities which made up her week previously, e.g., day centre, art, cooking, socialising, hairdresser etc.

A further circle around the perimeter would constitute the activities she was participating in now and what she would like to spend time doing. From this we would identify what was needed in order to facilitate her participation. She found spending so much time with Harry strange, as they had always led busy independent lives, although she was reluctant to go anywhere alone. We discussed how she could do things without Harry once she had harnessed support from the group she was joining, e.g., sharing lifts, or using a mobility scooter in the summer.

We talked about her low mood, and I put her in touch with an SLT who was also a trained a counsellor. Babs had stopped taking antidepressants, feeling reluctant about medication, but acknowledged that her mood was 'difficult to manage'. She had attended a coffee morning at the church – she was the only attendee; she joined the catholic WI to make friends but continued to feel isolated and lonely. Nobody from the church came to visit. Harry put up a sign in the local post office trying to set up a coffee morning for people who had survived a stroke but gained no interest.

17/1/08 Post-therapy assessment

Cinderella lives in a house where 2 stepsisters and her stepmother she disliked her family she worked in the house. The postman delivered the invitations of the ball to the palace. The stepsister was so excited that the invitation. Cinderella was not included, she sweeped up the floor. The fairy came to the rescue she waved the wand and Cinderella was changed to a beautiful girl. Cinderella went to the ball. The prince danced with her. At midnight she went home in the coach. The next day the Prince came round with a shoe. He tried the stepsister's foot – no! The prince came round to Cinderella – yes! The wedding of the Prince and Cinderella happened.

Palpa 3.1 Sentence Comprehension – silent thinking pauses for planning. Phrases punctuate naturally due to cohesive predicate structure.
Verbs (15) Nouns (16)

CIAT verbs 28/30: Using take/put spontaneously and accurately in sentences now.

Babs's language assessment demonstrated clear improvements in language processing, word retrieval and sentence formation. Babs was gaining accuracy and speed in her practised CIAT words, with 100% fluent production in one of her final sessions.

A friend commented on her progress. Her use of prepositional phrases which were once problematic started to improve once verb arguments became more consistent. Babs could now create a passive construction from an active sentence if given plenty of time. She had taken the train to London on her own and was met by her daughter en route for a day out together.

In spite of her linguistic gains, Babs left our time together feeling very low. I had not supported Babs and her family adequately through a process of adjustment and discussion around depression. I believe she did not take up the counselling sessions offered by a different therapist, and lost touch with her.

References

Armstrong, A. and Ferguson, A. (2010) Language, meaning, context, and functional communication, *Aphasiology*, 24(4): 480–496.

Beeke, S., Beckley, F., Johnson, F., Heilemann, C., Edwards, S., Maxim, J. and Best, W. (2015) Conversation focused aphasia therapy: Investigating the adoption of strategies by people with agrammatism. *Aphasiology*, 29(3): 355–377.

Brady, M. C., Kelly, H., Godwin, J., Enderby, P. and Campbell, P. (2016) Speech and language therapy for aphasia following stroke. *Cochrane Database Systematic Review*, Jun;1(6).

Caplan, D. (1987) *Neurolinguistics and Linguistic Aphasiology. An Introduction*. Cambridge Studies in Speech Science and Communication. Cambridge University Press.

Chapey, R., Duchan, J., Elman, R. J., Garcia, L. J., Kagan, A., Lyon, J. G. and Simmons-Mackie, N. (2000). Life participation approach to aphasia: A statement of values for the future. *ASHA Leader*, 5: 4–6.

Conroy, P., Sage. K. and Lambon-Ralph, M. A. (2009) Errorless and errorful therapy for verb and noun naming in aphasia. *Aphasiology*, 23(11): 1311–1337.

Difrancesco, S., Pulvermüller, F. and Mohr, B. (2012). Intensive Language-Action Therapy (ILAT): The methods. *Aphasiology*, 26: 1–35.

Egorova, N., Shtyrov, Y. and Pulvermuller, F. (2013) Early and parallel processing of pragmatic and semantic information in speech acts: Neurophysiological evidence. *Frontiers in Human Neuroscience*, 7: 86.

Egorova, N., Pulvermüller, F. and Shtyrov, Y. (2014) Neural dynamics of speech act comprehension: an MEG study of naming and requesting. *Brain Topography*, 27(3): 375–392.

Egorova, N., Shtyrov, Y. and Pulvermüller, F. (2016) Brain basis of communicative actions in language. *NeuroImage*, 125: 857–867.

Enderby, P. (2004). Making speech pathology practice evidence-based: Is this enough? *Advances in Speech-Language Pathology*, 6: 125–126.

Goldstein, K. (1948). *Language and Language Disturbances: Aphasic Symptom Complexes and Their Significance for Medicine and Theory of Language*. Grune & Stratton.

Holland, A. (1979) 'Some practical considerations in aphasia rehabilitation'. In M. Sullivan and M. Kommers (pp. 167–180). *Rationale for Adult Aphasia Therapy*. University of Nebraska Medical Center.

Jones E. V. (1986) Building the foundations for sentence production in a non-fluent aphasic. *Br J Disord Commun*. Apr;21(1): 63–82.

Kay, J., Coltheart, M. and Lesser, R. (1992) *Psycholinguistic Assessments of Language Processing in Aphasia*. Psychology Press.

Kleim, J. A. and Jones, T. A. (2008) Principles of Experience-Dependent Neural Plasticity: Implications for Rehabilitation After Brain Damage. *Journal of Speech, Language, and Hearing Research*, 51: S225–239.

Meinzer, M., Djundja, D., Barthel, G., Elbert, T. and Rockstroh, B., 2005. Long-term stability of improved language functions in chronic aphasia after constraint-induced aphasia therapy. *Stroke*, 36(7): 1462–1466.

National Service Framework for Older People (2001) Department of Health, UK. Available at: https://assets.publishing.service.gov.uk/government/uploads/system/uploads/attachment_data/file/198033/National_Service_Framework_for_Older_People.pdf

National Stroke Strategy (2007) Department of Health, UK. Available at: https://nsnf.org.uk/assets/documents/dh_081059.pdf

Patterson, K. and Shewell, C. (1987) 'Speak and spell: Dissociations and word class effects'. In M. Coltheart, G. Sartori and R. Job (Eds), *The Cognitive Neuro-psychology of Language* (pp. 273–294). Erlbaum.

Pound, C., Parr, S., Lindsay, J. and Woolf, C. (2000). *Beyond APHASIA: Therapies for Living with Communication Disability*, 1st edition. Routledge.

Pulvermüller, F., Neininger, B., Elbert, T., Mohr, B., Rockstroh, B., Koebbel, P. and Taub, E. (2001) Constraint-induced therapy of chronic aphasia after stroke. *Stroke*, 32: 1621–1626.

Royal College of Physicians (2008). *National Clinical Guideline for Stroke*, 3rd edition. Intercollegiate Stroke Working Party (ICSWP).

Sackett, D. L., Rosenberg, W. M., Gray, J. A., Haynes, R. B. and Richardson, W. S. (1996) Evidence based medicine: What it is and what it isn't. *BMJ*, Jan;13:312.

Simmons-Mackie N.N and Damico, J. S. (1996) Accounting for handicaps in aphasia: Communicative assessment from an authentic social perspective. *Disability and Rehabilitation*, 18(11): 540–549.

Tomasello, M., Carpenter, M., Call, J., Behne, T. and Moll, H. (2005) Understanding and sharing intentions: The origins of cultural cognition. *Behavioral and Brain Sciences*, 28(5): 721–727.

Wheelwright, P. (1968) *Metaphor and Reality*. Indiana University Press.

Whitworth, A., Webster, J. and Howard, D. (2005) *A Cognitive Neuropsychological Approach to Assessment and Intervention in Aphasia. A Clinicians Guide*. Psychology Press, Taylor and Francis Group.

Wittgenstein, L. (1956) *Remarks on the Foundations of Mathematics*. Blackwell.

Ylvisaker, M., Hibbard, M. and Feeney, T. (2006) LEARNet: A resource for teachers, clinicians, parents, and students by the brain injury association of New York State. Errorless Learning. [online] Available at: http://www.projectlearnet.org/tutorials/errorless_learning.html>

3 | A systems approach to aphasia therapy

People with aphasia are neglected in the community, in rehabilitation centres, and sometimes in hospitals too. This is my experience over 27 years, and it has changed very little with time. The longer-term needs of people living with aphasia in the community are ignored. Wray and Clarke (2017) looked at 32 qualitative studies in their systematic review and thematic synthesis, published in the *British Medical Journal*. They showed that stroke survivors with communication difficulties have ongoing difficulties in managing communication outside the home, maintaining social networks, creating meaningful roles and 'taking control and actively moving forward with life'.

It is easy to see how our conventional medical approaches may actually prevent people from feeling they are in control of their lives. Wray and Clarke concluded that wider psychosocial factors should be considered in the rehabilitation of people with post-stroke communication difficulties and treatment must be designed to help survivors to manage the unique psychosocial consequences of post-stroke communication difficulties. I would add the many brain injured people with aphasia from conditions other than stroke, to this group of people, but I would also suggest that this book offers an effective intervention for this population.

The value of elements of systemic philosophy to the speech and language therapist working with aphasia is discussed here. A unified approach to aphasia therapy is where the language therapy, regardless of the preferred model of intervention, forms an integral part of a systemic approach to aphasia.

A comprehensive holistic model of rehabilitation following acquired brain injury has been shown to be more effective than standard multi-disciplinary

DOI: 10.4324/9781003178613-3

team community rehabilitation. (Cicerone et al. 2011). This research has shown that clients who receive holistic neurorehabilitation are twice as likely to make significant gains in community functioning than standard rehabilitation, and that it is successful for many years post-injury. In addition, holistic approaches to rehabilitation were shown to improve functional independence, community reintegration and life satisfaction. In spite of this evidence, there are hardly any services in the UK that provide such a service. They are expensive but if they are likely to obtain better outcomes, they may save money in the longer term.

Psychology and/or neuropsychology are main features of holistic neurorehabilitation services. However, we know you are unlikely to access psychological care if you have aphasia, and even in these services PWA rarely have access to an SLT who specialises in aphasia, and mostly do not have any input from a clinical psychologist. In a book entitled the Brain Injury Rehabilitation workbook, which discusses holistic neurorehabilitation, there is no mention of aphasia, even in its index. This alone points to the limitations of services available to those with aphasia after brain injury.

Despite learning 20 years ago that psychotherapeutic groups help clients with normalisation and adjustment to disability and knowing that psychosocial disability is the best predictor of long-term service use, much more so than physical disability or cognitive disability (Hodgkinson et al. 2000), this knowledge has not translated into service provision.

Hodgkinson et al. (2000) also found that 6–17 years post-injury, patients were still using services to assist with adjustment to disability and community integration. Klonoff et al. (2001) showed that higher ratings of staff and family relationships predicted better outcomes and productivity ats many as 11 years post-rehabilitation. The question I have, therefore, is why our clients with aphasia and their families are yet to benefit from such knowledge.

References to such groups in the context of psychology and disability were made many years ago by Rappaport (1987, 1995), who outlined the following three ways to empower individuals following injury:

- Work with individuals within their social context to prevent problems before they occur
- Clients often feel marginalised and oppressed. They require advocacy to effect change in the system
- Empowerment = increasing clients' sense of autonomy and self-determination enabling them to represent their interests in a responsible way

In Chapter 7 I will be demonstrating that carefully designed aphasia cafes help facilitate normalisation of disability and adjustment for PWA, and how systemic approaches to such groups are a good substitute for psychotherapy.

Clinical psychologist and Auschwitz survivor, Edith Eger writes, 'The opposite of depression is expression' (Eger 2020). If this is the case, what happens to the PWA aphasia experiencing depression? How can the PWA manage to express, and to whom? We all know that it is psychologically helpful to discuss challenges in our lives, so why do we not *prioritise* assisting those with severe aphasia who are likely to be coping with associated depression, to reach some expression around this distress in order to reach some kind of healing? The answer is, we don't know how, so we avoid the problem and pretend it isn't there.

Ongoing trials of different types of therapy are surely no substitute for re-thinking and analysing what combination of therapy and intervention are going to be most helpful for people with aphasia. Current clinical practice operates out of disconnected approaches and isolated solutions whilst ignoring the wider picture, to the detriment of those who are suffering as they attempt to live with aphasia.

During a debate at the BAS Aphasia Therapy Symposium in 2017, it was reported that 45% of PWA feel abandoned with therapy being inadequate in terms of quantity. I wondered what they thought of the content of their therapy when they looked back on it some months and years later. It was suggested that substantial therapy is needed to make a different to stroke patients; however, in my view this does not consider that thinking about aphasia therapy differently might result in better use of therapy time such as it is. This chapter discusses why I believe systemic approaches to therapy might be the way to address some of these problems.

Prigatano (2013) and Wilson and Betteridge (2019) have promoted holistic neurorehabilitation for many years, where social and familial, as well as cognitive, language and physical difficulties are addressed in a unified manner by the multidisciplinary team for the maximum benefit of the client and family. A systemic approach further enhances this model of service delivery, as it benefits both staff, relatives and clients. Models such as the one pictured below, by way of example, are often used in formulating an overall view of the difficulties experienced by the person with a brain injury, in rehabilitation settings (Yeates et al. 2008)

An extremely useful model for understanding brain injury, this schema certainly helps clinicians to obtain and hold onto a holistic overview of the

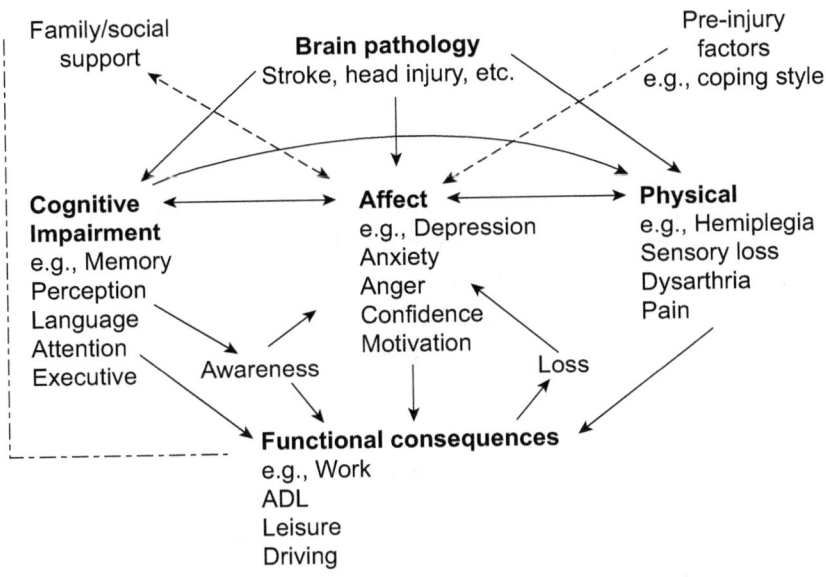

Figure 3.1 A biopsychosocial model of the impact of acquired brain injury

Source: Yeates et al. 2008

client. However, I would suggest such models do not give sufficient promi-nence to aphasia where *aphasia is the primary and overriding impairment.*

In other words, aphasia is very different in nature from cognitive-communication impairments, and the presence of aphasia would take on a more central role within a model that seeks to understand it as fully as pos-sible. Training of conversation partners and indeed staff in the skills required for communicating with PWA, is usually very limited in neurorehabilitation centres that can often focus more on other cognitive challenges. In many people with aphasia who also present with cognitive impairments early on, these aspects seem to recover at a different rate from the language, which can follow an altogether different timescale.

I was working in a centre for rehabilitation less than five years ago, where Mr. Bowen was residing following a left-sided MCA stroke, leaving him with 'no speech, and cognitive behavioural disorder', characterised by 'inappro-priate actions', according to the patient's notes. The SLT for the centre was not experienced with aphasia, had too many other clients to manage, and had been absent for some weeks at this time. There was much debate between his family and the clinical team about his returning home. His family were described to me by the team as 'a difficult family'. The clinical team had considered him unable to make his own decisions and therefore a DOLS (Deprivation of Liberty Safeguards) had been applied for.

In systemic terms, Mr. Bowen had received a 'totalising' clinical diagnosis (White and Epston 1990): cognitive behavioural disorder. Once a diagnosis is written down, it is hard for others or indeed the client and family, to see around it, question it, change it or even make room for progress and change! The words we use label the person as the problem and the problem as inherent to the person (e.g., victim, incoherent, mute, non-compliant, aggressive, unmotivated are a few sad examples I come across). Using labels absolves us from any responsibility towards the client to meet them where they are and to fully understand their experience.

An untrained rehabilitation assistant who is told a client has 'cognitive-behavioural disorder', will naturally approach that person with an element of caution and apprehension, rather than warmth and openness. We all as humans immediately sense and react to the stance adopted by others when we see them; the person with aphasia is no different. Difficulty accessing language does not mean social awareness is impaired. It was instantly clear to me that Mr. Bowen was experiencing moderate receptive and severe expressive aphasia with additional dyspraxia. This latter difficulty interfered with his ability to gesture and point effectively, leading to misinterpreted or 'inappropriate' gestures – terms which 'fitted' with the original diagnosis of cognitive behaviour disorder.

Through the use of drawing and writing, facial expression and gesture, I confirmed that he was extremely frustrated at not being heard or understood. He was frightened and angry, because he knew he was being treated as someone without mental capacity to make any decisions and was on the way to a nursing home (prematurely) for elderly residents! Aphasia had not been considered when deciding his mental capacity. I challenged the DOLS decision because I felt it had huge ethical ramifications and influenced whether or not he had a say in where he would live and who would control his finances. I talked to the family and found them to be extremely loving and wanting the best for their father. I then demonstrated with staff how I interacted with Mr. Bowen using supported conversation.

Eventually, the mental capacity assessment was repeated, Mr. Bowen chose to return home with care and authorised his son to handle his finances; his 'behaviour' resolved in the centre, not surprisingly. Such a case will not be a surprise to many SLTs. However, aspects of my systemic training enabled me to consider wider issues, such as my own stance in relation to his family, the staff, my own feelings about his situation, as well as hearing about how he had devotedly nursed his mentally ill wife alone for 40 years. She had died shortly before his stroke and he was grieving the loss of her, his role in caring for her, the relationship they had before she was ill, and many other factors that were feeding into his distress and not being addressed. One of his sons had committed suicide, and the rest of the family were bound by grief for him as well as for their mother, and yet no one had heard these stories before choosing to 'diagnose' the family as 'difficult'.

Mr Bowen, because of having aphasia, had received no mental health support whatsoever for the bereavement of his wife and for the bereavement associated with the loss of his ability to communicate; in fact, one could say he was just presented with further obstacles to negotiate. As Lynn Hoffmann, family therapist states 'Therapy in the medical model operates from a distance, assumptions are blaming and judgemental. This hiatus makes it limiting in how much the family can move on' (Hoffman 1990). The power of health workers is far-reaching and can be very destructive; I believe systemic therapy can goes a long way to prevent and redress this.

'Philosophy' has already been used frequently in this book and so it would seem right to afford it some kind of explanation here. After all, systemic thinking could be viewed as a philosophy about life. Philosophy is the 'love of wisdom' and wisdom 'the ability to use your knowledge and experience to make good decisions and judgments' (Cambridge English Dictionary 2021). The word therapist derives from the ancient Greek to mean to 'serve' or 'medically treat' without using drugs or surgery, suggesting the body is able to restore itself to a certain extent. The work of the therapist, one would deduce, is to provide an environment which is conducive to such recovery. This makes it distinct from conventional medicine, where treatment is expected to be restorative. Increasingly, however, we are seeing that some personal responsibility for lifestyle by the individual is required in order for medication to be effective and hopefully preventative.

Primary care has been moving towards a patient focussed treatment model, rather than the traditional view that the patient is a passive recipient of a doctor's 'medicine' and is 'done to' by the practitioner. For example, self-management (NHS England and NHS Improvement) is focussed on helping people with long term conditions to develop the knowledge, skills and confidence they need to manage their own health care effectively so that they are less heavily dependent on services that may or may not be able to meet their needs.

How this is achieved is not spelled out, however. One cannot expect patients to change their perspective on this without feeling 'abandoned' in some way by the healthcare system. Systemic approaches to therapies put the client very much in charge of their therapy by altering the balance of power, as we shall see. They present therapy in such a way that the client can see and reach for agency in their lives. When we consider this in the light of Wray and Clarke's work, referenced above, we can hope for a way to start out in the way we mean to go on.

Narrative therapy in systemic terms, and all that accompanies it (White 2007), fits well with the current notion of self-management; as it encourages us to see that the person is not the problem; the problem is the problem, and we have some choice about the stories we tell about our experiences.

Systemic therapy is often viewed as a form of 'counselling' therapy, hence its predominance in mental health settings. I have heard SLT's remark that a systemic approach is a counselling approach 'rather than' speech therapy. I disagree with this, but the view does not surprise me; it is not easy to explain in a short space of time.

As already described, PWA mostly do not access psychological support; such support is entirely dependent on an ability to comprehend and express language; the very thing that is impaired! In 27 years of aphasia therapy, I have met just one clinical psychologist who is interested in directly support- ing the client with aphasia and willing to learn some tools with which to do so. This is not a criticism of psychologists, rather a factor which further illus- trates the need for the speech and language therapist to better understand their own and others' family systems and identities in order to provide the necessary support in the context of their work with people with Aphasia and seek further support from psychology where needed.

Health-related quality of life (HRQL) measures are used to help us understand the impact of disease or disability on a person's life and to measure the effectiveness of intervention. Research studies that have looked at HRQL in people with mild or moderate aphasia report that reduced HRQL is associated with low psychological well-being and depression, reduced activity levels and high levels of communication disability (Hilari and Byng 2001). Quality of life assessment for people with severe aphasia is relatively neglected, and my experience shows that PWA which is severe do not access mental health support. Extensive research on the subject of health related quality of life in people with severe aphasia continues to be carried out, but I will be suggesting that *systemic* approaches that form an intrinsic part of aphasia therapy can help to address this in the longer term and provide meaningful data on this population in the future.

Providers of psychological therapies do not normally have the aphasia therapy skills with which to work with the client. Many years ago, I worked in a large well-known teaching hospital rehabilitation unit, where the very experienced clinical psychologist 'didn't see people with aphasia' because of the aphasia. Psychologists are often very stretched to support those with intact language after brain injury, let alone those with aphasia. I have rarely encountered clinical neuropsychologists who are interested in working with aphasia. In many instances SLTs are trying to do their best, some with extra counselling qualifications, some using the stepped care approach introduced in 2011, some with access to psychology for joint sessions. The majority of SLTs feel ill-equipped to support people psychologically through this huge life-changing event, and will talk about professional boundaries as if there is an invisible line to be drawn.

Anderson and Goolishian (1988) observed in their family work that men tend to value independence, autonomy and control, whereas women place the greatest value on relationship and connection. My subjective experience is that the majority of PWA aphasia that I have worked with have been male. Men have seemed to want to resolve the aphasia first and foremost in order to resume social family roles they previously held, whereas women can be quicker to see that they will need to adapt to living with the condition. Of course, this is a gross generalisation for which there will be many exceptions. However, I do believe that for men of an older generation, the sense of shame and psychological distress is not addressed when they also have aphasia. I will be exploring this further with reference to self-compassion and brain injury later in this book.

We are just beginning to see the use of systemic practice within healthcare; I trained alongside health visitors, NHS social workers, occupational therapists and psychologists. Two other speech and language therapists who work with adults with acquired brain injury and who are systemically trained have both published chapters referencing its use in clinical communication settings (Meredith and Yeates 2020; Prince 2017). Previous publications have touched on, but not been explicit about, systemic approaches and aphasia (Pound et al. 1999). As a clinician who has supervised many students and graduates of speech therapy training, I know this is yet to even begin to translate into training and practice. However, with the growth of systemic training in social work and related fields, I would expect these ideas to be relevant for our profession to consider for many years to come.

Research studies that have looked at evidence for speech therapy input versus no speech therapy, or speech therapy versus 'conversations with a non-SLT' (e.g., ACT NoW Study 2013) spark off fury amongst SLT colleagues who understandably, feel that that their work is somehow being misrepresented and its validity put in question. In our culture in Britain, stroke, brain injury and aphasia are still seen as problems to be remediated through treatments.

If we were to look at the evidence for 'systemic' approaches with aphasia therapy on the other hand, we would see new things. Firstly, it provides the therapist with a meta-awareness of what is taking place in the interaction, and how it is taking place. Therapists would learn the kinds of questions that will elicit meaningful answers from the client and become skilled at shaping the interactions in such a way that the client is very much in the driving seat of their therapy. They know that interactions in the 'hospital phase' of therapy may be very different from those that take place later on in the community. (A patient may report things as being 'really useful' in hospital, only to complain about them when they are still living with aphasia on their return home weeks or months later.) The 'when' is just as important as the 'what' and the 'who' and the 'how' in aphasia therapy.

After many years of attending aphasia and stroke conferences, I have the sense that researchers forge ahead, delving deeper and deeper into their own specific areas of interest, continuing to look for answers to the same kinds of questions. Whether the research is concerned with post- aphasia quality of life studies, or single word naming, or virtual reality, or semantic features, indeed any focussed field of study, there is a risk of confirmation bias, in my view, if they do not look to the wider picture of language and communication.

Rue and Snyder (1993) wrote about medical research:

> Like riding the merry-go-round, one chooses his horse. One can make believe his horse leads the rest. Then when a particular ride is finished, one must step off only to observe that the horse has really gone nowhere. Yet, it has been a thrilling experience. There may even be the yen to go again.

There can be a reluctance in our profession to see the range of interventions as spokes of a wheel which can all contribute to supporting the person with aphasia and their family.

I frequently hear the expression 'more research needs to be done in this area' when studies have not managed to come up with the clarity of data they hoped for. Increasingly I feel that less research in that area and alternative ways of thinking about it might be more helpful. Changing the question might be more useful in getting to an answer. Marcel Proust's *Remembrance of Things Past* comes to mind here: 'The real voyage of discovery consists not in seeking new landscapes but in having new eyes' (Proust 1929[1923]).

Systemic training provided me with new eyes; I learned how to interchangeably apply different lenses to what I was dealing with both professionally and personally. I saw different value in what I was already doing and tried new ideas that I hadn't thought of before. It helped me to see that 'Therapy is not a treatment the client receives; the therapist gives or even offers, but rather an ongoing collaborative dance' (McDermott and Jago 2001).

Attitudes to disability have undeniably changed over the years since I qualified as an SLT. We talk about hearing impairment, Asperger's syndrome, visual impairment, to name but a few, as variations of 'normal'. This is thanks to a more holistic approach which demands tolerance and a responsibility for society itself to reduce the handicap associated with such impairments.

I would argue, however, that where many impairments are easily 'understood', such as hemiparesis or deafness, aphasia is not visible; it is hard to understand, and it presents differently in each person. It takes time to understand and grasp what the person with aphasia is trying to adjust to. More than twenty years have passed, and I still don't understand aphasia fully; indeed, what I have become surer of, is the sheer diversity and complexity of aphasia; its ability to surprise, to restore, to be compensated for and to confound. I also never cease to be amazed by the resilience of people and their families who experience such potential devastation of their life plans and find ways of forging ahead with hope.

Aphasia can be highly variable; it is affected by fatigue, social demands, worry, and multiple other human factors. People require resources to deal with this variability and tools for thinking about what is happening to them in a useful way. To return to the 'merry-go-round' analogy, we as aphasia therapists need to pick up the whole carousel, and take it to our clients, looking together at ways we can weave a story from those separate horses and combine them in the most effective way. A systemic approach does this. It takes static 'horses' which are not versatile and together with the

49

client creates a therapeutic relationship that makes them move through the process of therapy to a place of living better with aphasia.

When a family member experiences aphasia following a brain injury, the whole 'family' is affected and goes through a major life transition. Clients have to negotiate those changes with their loved ones, and in the absence of their complete language system. We all experience role re-negotiation through life, when we start a new job, become a parent, are made redundant, children leave home, we retire, lose a parent etc. Roles change in aphasia; the nearest and dearest have to try and accommodate these changes, and previous coping strategies in the face of difficulty may no longer be effective, particularly if such strategies depend on a communication style which has fundamentally altered.

Family therapists view families as dynamic, evolving entities. Put simply (and this is not by any means a complete description of the subject), families have to live within social cultural and spiritual expectations; they develop their own ways of jointly negotiating decisions as a group, and each family member has their own set of personal beliefs influenced by interactions outside the family (Dallos and Draper 2010). Furthermore, families tend to operate out of beliefs about power, intimacy and boundaries, rules and tasks, as well as gender. A family needs to be able to adapt and restructure so that it can go on functioning; if they respond too rigidly to stress, then unhealthy patterns of behaviour can occur (Dallos and Draper 2010). Family therapy can help these difficult processes to take place. Aphasia families can benefit from such approaches, delivered by aphasia-trained SLTs, to support re-negotiation within the family to living with aphasia at different points along the process of recovery.

No doubt SLTs will recognise that those clients and or families who find it easier to discuss, problem solve and reflect in the face of adverse circumstances often adapt more successfully to change than those who don't. Sometimes a client's reporting of a situation may be very different from a spouse's version of events. What can be said in the therapy room cannot necessarily be said in front of the partner; not through dishonesty, but merely through a desire to protect one another. That is what families do. Some families increase their rigidity in the face of pressure as a coping mechanism, and distress and conflict arise. Families cope better if they can 'respond flexibly to changing circumstances and are able to change their rules and maps to fit the new situation' (Burnham 1999).

As a systemically trained SLT, or as a family therapist, the therapist learns to be more curious about the family/relationship/historical dynamics, to ask questions, re-evaluate their understanding of the situation constantly and involve the PWA and their family and environmental 'context'. In this way, families can be helped to respond more flexibly in the face of their distress.

The main principles of the Milan structural family therapists, which are hypothesising, circularity and neutrality, have helped me to adopt a more neutral and accepting stance in the face of difficulties (Cecchin 1987; Boscolo et al. 1987). Jones (1986) advocated hypothesis-forming in aphasia therapy. Hypothesis means 'a supposition or proposed explanation made on the basis of limited evidence as a starting point for further investigation' (OUP 2021). Psycholinguistic assessment of language might raise hypotheses about where the level of language breakdown might be. The therapist's job is to test these hypotheses through 'diagnostic therapy' and find the one that best fits the given presentation of the PWA.

Similarly, social constructionist approaches to systemic therapy adopt hypothesising as a way of thinking about the wider context of clients and their situations. In some clinical settings, therapists will already be familiar with the idea of formulation as a kind of hypothesis testing. One of the better-known Milan family therapists, Cecchin (1992) described the hypothesis as a 'way to contribute to the construction of a therapeutic relationship, creating a resonance with those involved, not a step towards discovering the "real" story'. Clinically we are often too intent on finding out the 'facts', as if there is one truth to be found, when in fact humans and language are highly complex and nebulous subjects. If we focus too quickly on the 'correct answer', as if it exists, this is the moment when we stop being curious. The moment we stop being curious about our clients and their stories is the moment we stop opening up new possibilities for the client and their family.

There are several aspects of hypothesising that make it a useful approach for aphasia therapy intervention:

Hypothesising helps therapists to connect behaviours of family members in a useful way, and to generate useful explanations of the client's context as a totality (Tomm 1985). Carl Tomm was also an advocate for circular ways of thinking rather than lineal which will be explained more in Chapter 5.

Hypothesising draws attention to the therapeutic relationship, to the context of the referring agency, and the agency in which the therapist works.

Hypothesising helps to keep ideas flowing, giving authority to the client and family, who become experts on their own life contexts.

Finally, creating and re-creating hypotheses avoids blame and shame (more on this later) – it offers up possibilities, none of which are attributable to one person's behaviour. Rather, it shines a spotlight on the interactive and recursive nature of our interpersonal relationships, rather than on any one individual.

Cecchin (1987) was keen that the therapist might highlight, through their hypothesis forming, the right amount of 'difference' in their (tentatively offered) suggestion from the explanation that the family might be holding that is causing them difficulty. (Robert had been the disciplinarian in the family. When he lost his spoken language, it was presumed that he could no longer hold this role within the family setting. As a result, family members avoided conversations with him, and he felt excluded. Exploring the idea that he might be able to communicate his wishes differently regarding his children's behaviour, and allowing space for him to do so, enabled him to regain an aspect of his family life that was important to him.)

Cecchin also asked therapists to avoid the verb 'to be' when describing a person's behaviour. For example, 'he is depressed' suggests a state of affairs that is more static than 'he is behaving as if he is depressed', in the minds of both family and therapists. If we as therapists start to use less totalising language, being aware that language can create reality, we can begin to be more open to alternative scenarios and develop a sense of optimism together with our clients.

Language forms reality

Information gathering for the aphasia therapist might involve creating hypotheses around a person's behaviour, their thoughts and their emotional experience and how these might interrelate (Papp 1983). It helps close others to think more widely about the experience for the person with aphasia, but also the reverse, where the PWA might need some encouragement to see the perspective of the family member/friend.

From an overview of the skills that systemic training aims to develop, below, it will be seen that many of these are highly desirable in the work of the aphasia therapist: indeed, I have found such skills invaluable to my work. Whether the aphasia therapist is offered the chance to adequately develop such skills within their own profession remains doubtful:

- An ability to co-create a therapeutic alliance with each person in the therapy room
- An ability to develop systemic hypotheses with clients and co-workers, using them to inform their questioning
- An ability to maintain a stance of curiosity throughout a session
- An ability to use circular questions to make connections and distinctions
- An ability to discuss practice to make links with theory, so that theory becomes 'lived practice' and practice becomes 'lived theory'
- Ability to consider different ethical postures, showing understanding that language creates social realities
- Able to work as a member of a therapeutic team and show self and relational reflexivity with awareness of the GRACES
- Demonstrate use of feedback from clients, colleagues and supervisor to inform practice
- Ability to use supervision to develop personally and professionally

'It is the specific way of asking questions that defines the stance of the systemic therapist and it is the specific stance systemic therapists assume in relation to their clients that allows them to generate these questions' (Rivet and Street 2009).

Questions are 'circular' because they are suggested by client's responses (Cronen 1995). The therapist expands the client's response by asking the next question, by relating it to other time-frames, other people, or consequences. The aim is to elicit ideas, create contexts for others, think about who speaks and who doesn't, different time frames, who is addressed and who isn't, formation of relationships, formation of trust, respect, collaboration, conflict, and so on. It is not hard to see why these approaches seem to fit with working with aphasia.

Aphasia therapy sessions are traditionally planned in advance, however latterly I have only planned a small part of the session, as this makes it easier to be responsive to what the client is bringing on that particular day and authentically position myself more collaboratively with the client.

De Shazer's Brief Therapy view that 'the key is utilising what the client brings with him to meet his needs in such a way that the client can make a satisfactory life for himself' resonates with me in the context of aphasia, as does the idea that 'no matter how awful and complex a situation is, a small change in one person's behaviour can make profound and far-reaching differences in the behaviour of all persons involved' (De Shazer 1985). This can be applied to changes in a family's communication style and environment. It can also be used in supporting the person with aphasia to adopt their own way of educating others as to the nature of their aphasia and what is needed to circumvent the problems that it can create.

A systemic view might ask the question about power – is it taken by others or are we sometimes responsible for giving the power to others, even when it leads to our own suffering?

Communication is not just about transmitting a message. The Latin derivation suggests 'making common' and is linked to the notions of commune and community. Social constructionists such as Cronen (1995), state that 'we communicate, therefore we are'. The power of language, however, is such that in creating one picture of reality through language, it pre-disposes us to see reality in that way rather than in all the other ways in which we might have understood events (Cronen1995).

We cannot **not** respond or express (Watzlawick et al. 1967). Silence is a response, and one that I don't think we use enough as aphasia therapists. At the risk of sparking controversy, I would say that SLTs have a tendency to enjoy talking! I have become increasingly aware that the times when I have paused, or struggled with what to say next, is often the time the client starts to communicate or brings in something unexpected which creates new opportunities in therapy.

The systemic notion that 'a problem system is always a linguistic system . . . problems do not have an objective existence in and of themselves but only through conversation with others' (Anderson and Goolishian 1988) prompts us as aphasia therapists to think differently about how those conversations about issues face by PWA may be conducted in more useful ways.

Rehabilitation assistants, health care assistants, and similar health workers find it difficult to work with someone with aphasia. They are often afraid to offend, to lose face, and often feel this sense of fear to be due to their own incompetence or inadequacy in some respect. If trained SLTs are unsure about working with aphasia, how can we expect untrained workers to do so? Supported conversation training is essential, but it is not the whole story. Systemic approaches help us to consider these wider contexts, acknowledge uncertainty and doubt, and offer a wider and more comprehensive web of support to our assistants, without whom we are so limited in what we can achieve therapeutically.

In terms of managing an NHS aphasia caseload management in community settings, I found that a systemic approach uncovered wider benefits, such as reducing waiting lists, minimising distress, increased satisfaction of clients and their families and a new sense of autonomy for me as the clinician as well as for the client in therapy.

Case: Andrew

Andrew was a 54-year-old married man with two sons who both lived away from home. Andrew had a very demanding job in local government. He was a keen runner, which he still managed to fit around working a 75-hour working week in the office.

When I first met Andrew, he had been waiting a few minutes, before dashing into the room very fast, smiling and saying breathlessly, as he pulled a chair up to the table 'yes this….it's what I need . . . get my words . . . now . . . now . . . it was 2 no 3 no 4 weeks . . . I was in hostelit . . . all the time . . . '. Andrew's demeanour was energetic, friendly and very restless. The aphasia was characterised by word finding difficulty, hesitations, and dysfluency at word initial positions. Auditory comprehension was difficult to assess and presented very variably as he had difficulty stopping to listen, let alone think clearly. Andrew struggled to find the right words and often used the wrong word, which he was sometimes aware of often he wasn't.

He was asking me to 'fix' the problem as it was 'already 4 weeks' since his stroke, which happened while he was out running. He 'knew' from watching the television, that you 'have to act FAST when a stroke happens'. He took up running to keep fit so that he could avoid having a stroke and counterbalance the enormous responsibility his job entailed.

Previously, I might have felt an obligation to immediately carry out an in-depth language assessment and go with Andrew's expectations of working on his word finding difficulties and train the family in how to use supported conversation techniques with Andrew to help him to participate in conversations and retain his family role of father, husband, bread-winner and runner. I might have become frustrated that Andrew's wife did not want to take part in such training and felt critical that she appeared disinterested in that aspect of therapy.

Taking a systemic stance, I was first more curious about Andrew's presentation as being so rushed, so intent on a fix that he struggled to listen, let alone hear what I had to say. I listened carefully to what he had to say and did not interrupt. Gradually, he slowed down and relaxed. I began to feel that Andrew's cultural values of hard work, success and effort could hamper his language recovery due to fatigue and processing overload. I suggested to him we try to establish a more useful way of interacting together.

First of all, I asked him to have a break from talking and to listen, while I addressed the 'Act FAST' advertisement by the Stroke Association. The acronym refers to the need to act quickly when there is sudden facial weakness, arm weakness, and speech problem, so that specialist treatment for the circulation problem causing the stroke can be obtained as soon as possible. I have met many people with aphasia, who, after the acute phase of hospitalisation and possible thrombolysis (clot busting treatment), firmly believe that if their speech is affected, the urgency for aphasia treatment is still there. Whilst I would advocate speech and language support as early as possible for the family, the client is often unable to process what has happened for some time while physiological recovery is taking place. Aphasia therapy will be ongoing over a period of time.

Secondly, I told Andrew, as I often do when I see people for the first time, that he was unlikely to regain his speech 100% to the same level of efficiency as before the stroke, but that together we would aim to him to get as close to this as possible. This was not to remove hope for Andrew; quite the contrary. Janine Roberts (2005) refers to unspoken things 'taking on a growing presence, we choose to hear, ignore or silence stories and this shapes our identities'. It is a way of being transparent with what I know as a speech and language therapist, regardless of what false promises or indeed totalising doom-laden predictions (e.g., 'if you haven't recovered in 6 months you never will') he may have received during his brief inpatient stay. A systemic approach is a collaborative one. Furthermore, a systemic view is one that embraces the fluidity of life, we are all continuously changing and 'on the way' to living a better life. Progress after aphasia continues for many years as people and circumstances change to find new ways of interacting and finding purpose in life.

We embarked on semantic language therapies for word finding, reading therapy at sentence and later paragraph levels, incorporating strategies for slowing down, identifying fatigue, and later writing short pieces and self-editing his work. Andrew described his speech as having 'traffic jams'. His analogy was used to talk about ways to reduce traffic jams (slowing the traffic) and he started to apply this to his speech, resulting in greater fluency and a calmer demeanour. Previous automatic strategies of working harder and faster backfired in language and speaking: his speech deteriorated, and he became angry and frustrated with himself. I asked him if there are some things of value that require waiting for, rather than working at.

This aphasia therapy and language work was interspersed throughout with 'systemic' conversations. Andrew's story was one of being the son of a perfectionist father, who imposed aspirations that were never fully achievable; he was desperate to succeed here too, to recover from his stroke so that nothing would change; this way he would still be in 'control' of things.

We talked about family myths, views of 'success' and I asked Andrew why he would wish to return to a job that has made him so ill? How could he have noticed that he was becoming unwell? Did he notice when his employees were struggling with their health? What other things did he dream of doing in his life? How might one know when to reduce one's working hours? How do his sons view the situation?

Such conversations help to open up alternative stories, other than the one of success (returning to work full-time) versus failure (part-time return or not at all) which dominated Andrew's narrative at this time. In talking about how his laid-back second son enjoyed life more than his successful, but desperately anxious older son, Andrew began to form an idea of how he would like his future to be. Slowly he began to talk about how he might allow his wife to support him conversationally and how listening to her stories might throw a new light on what her life has been like in recent years. He reflected on the change and fear that the stroke had meant for his wife and sons, and how he might support them too through his recovery. He began to think about what not being back in his job would say about him to his family. This enabled him to take the perspective of others and to feel the gratitude that his family had for his survival and excellent recovery to date. Andrew talked about ways he and his wife might be able to allow space for alternative plans for the future, which might release constraints for both of them and make space for the joy to be had in life.

Andrew said to me after 12 weeks that he felt ready to stop therapy and spend more time at home, and to think about his next plans. He struck me as a calmer man, he was listening as well as speaking, and he had made excellent progress in terms of his language recovery. Furthermore, he felt sure there was plenty more language progress still to come. He had regained some control over his language and had the tools with which to progress further.

Ultimately, Andrew returned to a part time job on a lesser wage but only after taking several hiking trips with his anxious son in the Lake District, to 'teach him about what really matters in life and to do what I always wanted to be doing'.

References

ACT NoW Study (2013) Trial participants' experiences of early enhanced speech and language therapy after stroke compared with employed visitor support: A qualitative study nested within a randomized controlled trial. *Clinical Rehabilitation*, 27(2): 174–182.

Anderson, H. and Goolishian, H. A. (1988) Human systems as linguistic systems: preliminary and evolving ideas about the implications for clinical theory. *Family Process*, 27(4): 371–393.

Boscolo, L., Cecchin, G., Hoffman, L. and Penn, P. (1987). *Milan Systemic Family Therapy: Conversations in Theory and Practice*. Basic Books.

Burnham, J. (1999) Approach, Method, Technique: Making Distinctions and Creating Connections. from *Human Systems: The Journal of Systemic Consultation and Management*, 3(1): 3–26.

Cambridge English Dictionary (2021), Essential British English Dictionary Online. Available at: https://dictionary.cambridge.org/dictionary/essential-british-english/ (accessed 29 July 2021).

Cecchin, G. (1992) 'Constructing therapeutic possibilities'. In S. McNamee, and K. J. Gergen (Eds), *Therapy as Social Construction* (pp. 86–95). Sage.

Cecchin, G. (1987) Hypothesising, circularity and neutrality revisited: An invitation to curiosity. *Family Process*, 26(4): 405–414.

Cicerone, K. D., Langenbahn, D. M., Braden, C., Malec, J. F., Kalmar, K., Fraas, M., Felicetti, T., Laatsch. L., Harley, J. P., Bergquist, T., Azulay, J., Cantor, J., Ashman, T. (2011) Evidence-based cognitive rehabilitation: Updated review of the literature from 2003 through 2008. *Arch Phys Med Rehabil*. Apr;92(4): 519–530. doi:10.1016/j.apmr.2010.11.015 PMID: 21440699

Cromwell, Rue L. and Snyder, C. R. (1993) *Schizophrenia: Origins, Processes, Treatment and Outcome*. Oxford University Press.

Cronen, V. E. (1995). Coordinated management of meaning: The consequentiality of communication and the recapturing of experience. The consequentiality of communication, pp.17–65.

Dallos, R. and Draper, R. (2010) *An Introduction to Family Therapy. Systemic Theory and Practice*. Third edition. McGraw-Hill Education.

De Shazer, S. (1985). *Keys to Solutions in Brief Therapy*. W. W. Norton.

Eger, E. (2020) *The Gift: 12 Lessons to Save Your Life*. Ebury Publishing.

Hilari, K. and Byng, S. (2001) Measuring quality of life in people with aphasia: The Stroke Specific Quality of Life Scale. *Int J Lang Commun Disord.* 36: Suppl: 86–91. doi: 10.3109/13682820109177864 PMID: 11340850

Hodgkinson, A., Tate, R., Veerabangsa, A., Maggiotto, S. (2000) Measuring psychosocial recovery after traumatic brain injury: Psychometric properties of a new scale. *The Journal of Head Trauma Rehabilitation,* Vol. 14.

Hoffman, L. (1990) Constructing realities: An art of lenses. *Family Process,* Mar;29(1): 1–12.

Jones, E. V. (1986) Building the foundations for sentence production in a non-fluent aphasic. *Br J Disord Commun.* Apr;21(1): 63–82.

Klonoff, P. S., Lamb, D. G. and Henderson, S. W. (2001)Outcomes from milieu-based neurorehabilitation at up to 11 years post-discharge. *Brain Injury,* 15(5).

McDermott, I. and Jago, W. (2001) *Brief NLP Therapy.* Sage Publishing.

Meredith, K. H. and Yeates, G. N.(Eds) (2020) *Psychotherapy and Aphasia Interventions for Emotional Wellbeing and Relationships.* Routledge.

Oxford University Press (2021) *Definition of hypothesis* [online]. Available at https://www.lexico.com/definition/hypothesis (accessed 29 July 2021).

Papp, P. (1983) *The Process of Change.* Guilford Publications.

Pound, C., Parr, S., Lindsay, J. and Woolf, C. (1999) *Beyond Aphasia: Therapies for Living with Communication Disability.* Speechmark Editions.

Prigatano, G. (2013) Challenges and opportunities facing holistic approaches to neuropsychological rehabilitation. *Neurorehabilitation,* July;32(4):751–759.

Prince, L. (2017) Working with families after brain injury. In R. Winson, B. Wilson and A. Bateman (Eds) *The Brain Injury Rehabilitation Workbook.* The Guilford Press.

Proust, M. (1929[1923]) *Remembrance of Things Past,* Volume V, *The Captive (La Prisonnière).* Translated by C. K. Scott Moncrieff (revised by T. Kilmartin, 1981). Chatto and Windus.

Rappaport, J. (1987) Terms of empowerment/exemplars of prevention: Toward a theory for community psychology. *American Journal of Community Psychology,* 15(2): 121–148.

Rappaport, J. (1995) Empowerment meets narrative: Listening to stories and creating settings. *American Journal of Community Psychology,* 23(5): 795–807.

Rivett, M., and Street, E. F. (2009) *Family Therapy. 100 Key Points and Techniques.* Routledge.

Roberts, J. (2005) Transparency and self-disclosure in family therapy: Dangers and possibilities. *Family Process,* March;44(1): 45–65.

Tomm, C. (1985) 'Circular interviewing: A multi-faceted clinical tool'. In D. Campbell, and R. Draper (Eds), *Applications of Systemic Family Therapy.* Grune and Stratton.

Watzlawick, P., Beavin-Bavelas, J. and Jackson, D. (1967). Pragmatics of human communication: A study of interactional patterns, pathologies and paradoxes. W. W. Norton.

White, M. (2007) *Maps of Narrative Practice.* Norton Professional Books.

White, M. and Epston, D. (1990) *Narrative Means to Therapeutic Ends.* W.W. Norton.

Wilson, B. A. and Betteridge, S. (2019) *Essentials of Neuropsychological Rehabilitation.* Guilford Publications.

Wray, F. and Clarke, D. (2017) Longer-term needs of stroke survivors with communication difficulties living in the community: A systematic review and thematic synthesis of qualitative studies. *BMJ Open*, 7(10).

Yeates, G. N., Gracey, F. and Collicutt McGrath, J. (2008) A biopsychosocial deconstruction of 'personality change' following acquired brain injury. *Neuropsychological Rehabilitation*, 18(5–6): 566–589. doi:10.1080/09602010802151532

4 | The self of the therapist

Aphasia therapy requires a better understanding of identity than is currently available to SLTs, in my view. Language and identity are intricately entwined. The languages I speak and my cultural identity are inextricably entwined. The adage 'Know Yourself' has been a subject of interest for millenia. According to the ancient Greek, Pausanias, the saying was inscribed on the forecourt of the Temple of Apollo at Delphi, also known as the Oracle of Delphi. The ancient Chinese philosopher Lao Tzu wrote in his famous work, Tao Te Chung, 'Knowing others is intelligence. Knowing yourself is true wisdom.'

This chapter explains how an understanding of others first requires some understanding of the self. The therapist brings their own values, beliefs and experiences to the therapeutic relationship. Knowing why we are doing what we are doing is essential for active listening and active listening is one of the key underlying principles of successful therapy, both in counselling and, I would maintain, in aphasia therapy.

An 'ecological' approach considers how the therapist's view of the world, their way of talking, and their actions powerfully affect the therapeutic conversation and the client (Hedges 2005). We are usually unaware of this as we focus on the task in hand in therapy. Our own feelings relate to our specific gender, class, spiritual identity and personal stories and, I would argue, an awareness of the context we are operating out of is important if we are to be able to truly listen to the stories of our clients with aphasia.

Awareness means being sensitive to personal cultural issues and to think about how our own cultural identity influences understanding and acceptance of others who are like us and different from us. Such an awareness prepares us to be alert to how such factors may inhibit or promote the experience for each client that we meet. In presenting case examples of other

DOI: 10.4324/9781003178613-4

people's lives for this book, it is only right that I am prepared to represent my own case, as an aphasia therapist working systemically. I will attempt to show how, through systemic learning, I have learned who I am as an aphasia therapist, how I got there, and how this impacts on my work with clients with aphasia.

Whereas in conventional healthcare the professional is seen as separate from the patient, and aim to 'keep a professional distance', the systems view suggests that this is an illusion: an interaction between two people cannot take place without each of those people being affected in some way by the other. 'As we observe, we influence that which we are attempting to understand . . . . We do not discover behaviour, we create it' (Becvar and Becvar 1999).

During the 23 years I had already been working as a speech and language therapist and clinical educator, I became increasingly aware of a shift in my approach to my work with people with acquired communication disorders. However, I was having difficulty describing this to therapists I was trying to educate clinically. It appeared alien to their theoretical learning, which adopts a more 'first order' approach to therapy where the therapist 'gives', and the client 'receives'; or the supervising clinician 'teaches', and the student 'learns'. Of course, as mentioned earlier, clinical education requires a prescriptive approach initially, in order to provide the scaffolding on which to attach one's learning. From here, skills development can occur in a semi-structured manner.

My approach to working with aphasia is one I have developed gradually with experience. I found I was listening more and more to my 'patients', even adopting a slightly irreverent attitude to what I had been formally taught, being more interested in their views within their social and family context ('there is no meaning without context' (Bateson 1972)) and agreeing with them more than advising them on ways they should communicate. I sensed a shift in the power dynamic in the room, together with what started to feel like a more authentic relationship with the client in aphasia therapy sessions.

In retrospect, I had already begun to adopt a more second order cybernetic approach to my work 'together we create a shared understanding (Burnham 2005). De Shazer's view that 'the key is utilising what the client brings with him to meet his needs in such a way that the client can make a satisfactory life for himself' resonated with me, as did the idea that 'no matter how awful and complex a situation is, a small change in one person's behaviour can make profound and far-reaching differences in the behaviour of all persons involved' (De Shazer 1985). We as aphasia clinicians are not expected to provide all the answers; the answers lie within the therapeutic process.

I was drawn to systemic training as I felt I had more to learn about the complexities of communication in relation to particular clients and their families and was searching for new ways in which to think about the effects of disordered communication on people's lives and relationships.

Not only was I needing to clarify the way I was starting to work with PWA, but I needed to consider how to explain this approach to colleagues with sufficient theoretical support. Eventually I started to use the aforementioned 'circular questioning' style common to systemic practice with colleagues when trying to problem-solve or to find solutions to dilemmas relating to therapy. I noticed that they came up with better solutions when carefully worded questions enabled them to use their own resources as a starting point.

After my first session of systemic therapy training, which required self-reflection, I wrote: 'It feels strange to be so hesitant and have the time to reflect on ideas, but equally I realise the possible impact of the systemic approach on my own life and work might be greater than I was originally expecting.' This impact ended up bringing significant changes to my work, to the way I relate to clients and colleagues, as well as wider networks. Key areas of systemic theory included structural family therapy, coordinated management of meaning, narrative therapy and contexts of social difference (Dallos and Draper 2010) some of which are explored here.

My initial experience of systemic training was that I was waiting for direction from the tutors about what to learn and what to do next, (much like our clients with aphasia do when they come to see the SLT). After all, this is how I approached my undergraduate and postgraduate degrees.

This was not what happened. I learned about the importance of first knowing oneself, and really began to learn. Just as in SLT, it takes time and the development of a therapeutic relationship to share the balance of power in family therapy. Through experiencing techniques that family therapists use with families, I found I was able to form my own ideas about what to do next, within both my work and home life. Indeed, these ideas have prompted the writing of this book.

John Hill's genogram is a way of positioning the client and their family as the expert in their life and minimising the power of the therapist (Hills 2012) as we saw in the case study of Chapter 1. This key part of training, the compilation of a visual representation of three generations of one's family, helps us to understand what contributes to our own cultural identity, assumptions and stereotypes. Our own emotional triggers are culturally based, whether or not we happen to be aware of this. Our own unique cultural identity is well worth exploring, as it inevitably impacts on our therapeutic style and effectiveness. 'We belong to and move through a complex multiplicity of cultures' (Hardy and Laszloffy 1995).

'Culture' is a word that can mean many things; it covers gender, geography, race, religion, age, ability, appearance, class, ethnicity, education, employment, sexuality, sexual orientation and spirituality. Otherwise known as the 'social graces' (as developed by John Burnham 2013), these are meant to provide a framework within which to consider differences in other people and the contexts out of which they (and we) operate and communicate with one another.

Self-awareness on the part of the therapist is crucial in order to observe the therapeutic relationship we are building on with our clients. Our identity influences how we understand people who are of similar and different cultural backgrounds, and in order to actively listen to our clients we need to acknowledge that, just as your experience is unique, their experience is also unique. If a client brings up something that is culturally meaningful to us, we are emotionally affected by this, and really need to notice that, so that we don't inadvertently make ourselves the focus. The reverse is also true, in that we may make a reference or assumption that has far greater significance to the client, than it has for us. For example, insensitive assumptions about a client's literacy can induce feelings of shame that create an obstacle to the therapeutic relationship, even if they are not explicitly expressed.

Family therapists aim to be open to whatever is most significant to the client. When we look at a family genogram, we can see how transitions have altered families and family behaviours. The genogram reveals transitions and can be done at various times, to show how people reposition themselves, (or not) following change. Burnham (2013) claims that 'families are healthy if they can respond flexibly to changing circumstances and are able to change their rules and maps to fit the new situation'. This reference to the effects of significant transitional stages in the evolution of the family reminds us that our clients and their families face huge transitions following brain injury. With impaired or absent language, how do PWA and their families negotiate such transitions and what is the role of the SLT in facilitating this process? We often see brain injury in isolation, as one particular change that has happened in a family. However as human beings we all go through constant transitions. Starting work, parenting, the shifting sands of growing teenagers, bereavement, illness and so on. What are the resources we use to manage these transitions in our lives and what resources have our clients used in the past that demonstrate their ability to adapt to change and reorganise their lives?

Watts-Jones (2010) writes about the location of the therapist's self in therapeutic interactions to ensure that the therapist is considering their relationship with the client but also their relationship with the therapeutic relationship. He warns against inadvertent assumptions, such as not asking about things which may not be in your experience but might be significant for client. Further, there are times to share information with a client and times to hold back from doing so, and knowledge of one's own contexts can help to guide that decision, in my experience.

I once had an excellent student, very competent, who slightly lacked confidence in her clinical skills, as many students understandably do at this stage. I noticed that her sessions always concluded with her apologising profusely for 'not being very good' and hoping she had 'said the right things' to the client and family. Their response to this was invariably to console and reassure her and let her know how lovely she was. One could be forgiven for thinking the therapist was the client as they left the therapy room. I felt that she was seeking something from the therapeutic relationship that might not be so helpful to herself or the client in the longer term. I wondered how aware she was of this pattern.

Of course, it is right that the therapist should be able to acknowledge limitations in their experience, but also know how to discuss this uncertainty in a manner that is helpful to the client. A constant awareness of how the client feels the therapy is going is valuable to the therapist. Constantine and Kwan (2003) talk about therapist self-disclosure strengthening the therapeutic alliance and helping to bridge the gap in social power. They advocate that 'in the privileged position of therapist you should bear the initial vulnerability not the client' and say that clients find therapist disclosure reassuring and normalising, as it helps them to relate to the therapist therefore are more open in therapy.

I notice that with experience, I am ready to acknowledge difficulties as existing rather than trying to convince people they aren't there. It is ok to find things difficult and there is no easy answer – this has changed my approach and I have found that when you acknowledge this, clients are more likely to look for their own solutions collaboratively with you. I accept that it takes maturity and confidence to take calculated risks with clients to a certain extent, although all therapists can practice this to an extent within their own 'safety net' of knowledge.

In the context of my work with adults with acquired brain injury, a good example of therapist self-awareness is in the way we use our voices. The voice quality that we use in our interactions is necessarily formative and it influences the behaviour of others. It affects how someone perceives us, even though we might not even be aware of it. This is a good example of where I have applied knowledge learned through voice therapy training, to my work with PWA. Dr. Lesley Hendy, in her 5 Voices Training Progamme for teachers (www.the5voices.com/), demonstrates beautifully how using different voice qualities can positively influence the learning and behaviour of pupils. This principle applies to all contexts where communication takes place; not least the busy rehabilitation unit, which can be noisy and distracting, and even distressing places to be.

The loudness, pitch, harshness and rate of speech can instill a sense of either threat or reward in the person we are talking to. Research has demonstrated with the SCARF model (Rock 2008) that much of our motivation driving social behavior is governed by an overarching organising principle of minimising threat and maximising reward. SCARF stands for the five domains of experience (Status, Certainty, Autonomy, Relatedness and Fairness) which activate strong threats and rewards in the brain, thus influencing a wide range of human behaviours.

Following a brain injury, many clients are hypersensitive to noise, find it difficult to filter out extraneous sounds and can be overwhelmed by rapid, loud speech, even when well intentioned. I often work with rehabilitation assistants around becoming aware of their own voice use, so that they can make sure to appeal to the 'reward' system instead of the threat system of an already vulnerable client. Distressed clients, as well as those with complex cognitive communication challenges to overcome, often respond very differently to a calm, slow voice that gives them the message they are being supported, and reducing their fear, even if their comprehension is so severely impaired that they cannot decipher the words.

I have often seen nervous but well-intentioned clinicians masking their own uncertainty by using defensive voices, or even joking, with clients with aphasia, which, if not done with sensitivity, can put even greater distance between them and the client and allows little opportunity for the client to communicate their own position.

Systemic therapy requires self-reflection, so that we notice our responses to our clients and think about how our communication affects the client. Further, and this is especially important when working with PWA, we must explore what the client takes our words to mean and be interested in how what we say might affect them. We need to notice who might be included in the client's system, the resources the client is already using and be prepared to discard one therapy and try alternative ones, if we are being systemic.

Power and positioning

Discussion about the therapist self cannot continue without addressing concepts of power; a key term in systemic thinking, which has already been alluded to several times. Awareness of how we position ourselves and others in interactions is key to altering the balance of power and moving to a more authentic therapeutic relationship. Truly listening to our client with aphasia, which means sitting comfortably with silence, and just waiting, is one way to start to alter the power differential. You can't listen to others if your mouth is full of your own words (Hornstrup et al. 2012).

This is hard for 'professionals' to do, even if they are SLTs, as they are trained to be in the 'knowing' position, which seems to assume that this means 'informing' our clients. In fact, we can help them to inform us by protecting a silent space for them in which to find a way to initiate or reply. Communication is about doing as well as saying, and even silence is a response. As alluded to earlier, 'we cannot not respond or express' (Watzlawick et al. 1967).

Gale and Newfield (1992) weren't talking about aphasia when they said, 'The person with the greatest linguistic ability holds the greatest power.' However, nowhere is the imbalance of power more evident than in the aphasia vs non-aphasia interaction. This familiar imbalance led me to consider ideas about power in the clinical setting, and how I position myself as an aphasia therapist. Fredman (2007) says: 'People can be positioned by others or position themselves, e.g. as powerful or powerless, dominant or submissive, confident or apologetic, definitive or tentative, authorised or unauthorized.' Thinking consciously about how others might position us when we meet them should help us to meet our clients closer to where they are, rather than from our health worker position.

Positioning Theory is a social constructionist approach that first emerged in gender studies, talking about how men and women take up positions in discourses (Harré and Van Langenhove 1999). When we think about our own families and experiences, we can no doubt identify examples of where we have taken a position, ascribed it, contested it and even subverted the position we have been ascribed. In therapy, we assume a position, and this can alter according to whom we are talking, where we sit, the language we use, how and when we talk or listen, and what we ask of people. We bring with us discourses that have taken place in our lives outside our work context. Positioning is something that takes place dynamically, it is not static. 'Therapists need to be sensitive to the discourses that enter the therapy room' (Baum 2011).

Burnham (2005) talks about the therapist being transparent about the position taken in relation to talking in therapy (relational reflexivity), and how we take up certain identities and not others. I have found that through an exploration of discourses from my own life, I am much more aware of how these may impact positively or negatively on how I work with a client. I still have to be alert to these as they can influence how I am working without my being aware of it at times.

The same may be true for our clients. People differ in their willingness and/or their ability to position themselves and others. This will be referred to again later in Chapters 5 and 7. If we alter our position in the therapy room, it can encourage the client to alter theirs, although their capacity for this may be influenced by invisible social identity and educational factors too, for example how much power they would normally have within their own social network or relationships.

Vygotsky's question, 'Can we think without language? How are they related?' has always been very prominent for me in working with aphasia (Vygotsky 1962). I am perennially interested in ideas about 'thinking for speaking'. In aphasia, language itself (at a psycholinguistic level) can be impaired, as well as speech (articulatory), with or without additional cognitive processing difficulties. We who do not live with aphasia mostly have the language we need at our fingertips with which to position ourselves, but how is it for the person with aphasia without ready access to the language with which to either position themself, or contest, or subvert positions they have been ascribed, in the face of someone who has the power of language?

I run a weekly 'café' for people and their families who have aphasia. I am more aware now that I immediately position people when I introduce them (this is John, he is keen on motorbikes/had a stroke/is an artist etc). I ask them if they 'would like to get yourself a drink' (rather than would you like a drink), thereby expecting them to ask for something at the bar, by whatever means they can. I learned that members of the group position themselves and each other, in relation to me, their family members or carers as well as other professionals. I try to find the language or strategies by which to communicate with someone and support them to express themselves and position themselves too in the way they choose.

When I work with someone who is 'nonverbal', they can appear not to have access to their language system, either for understanding what is said or written, or for expressing themselves verbally. I have enormous power in positioning 'nonverbal' people in relation to me, and in relation to others present. Often, I am feeling my way, asking more questions, assuming things based on my previous experiences and asking the person if x or y is true for them or not. Consciousness of this extraordinary disadvantage for PWA is what makes me strive to find greater equality for them. People with significant cognitive deficits as a result of brain injury can still preserve a construct of 'selfhood' and carers play an important role in maintaining a positive selfhood for that person and positioning the self in discourse.

Transparency

Systemic therapists are often transparent about their method of work, beliefs, values and personal experinces in therapy, as a way of putting themselves on an equal, or collaborative level with the client (Roberts 2005). This helps them to be more aware of (a) what is being said in therapy sessions (for example narratives, beliefs, prejudices) (b) what is happening in therapy, (aphasia therapy activity) and (c) point out the things which may influence the therapeutic relationship (age, gender, race, culture,religion etc). There are many aspects of this that I have started to express in my work. I have found that 'disclosure' or 'transparency' can enhance the sense of autonomy for the client around their own therapy, and encourages them to look for their own strengths and resources.

Janine Roberts (2005) suggests guidelines for this by asking oneself certain questions about how we talk with clients. I have selected those which I use most, modifying some for the specific context of aphasia therapy rather than family therapy.

Is my desire to share theoretical beliefs and values that I have likely to be of interest, support, and use to my client? Or, am I wanting to show off to clients what I know?

Are there biases in models of therapy I am using that undermine the social identity of the client? (ie. education, literacy, gender) Am I using language about change that is respectful of the clients and connects to their language?

Be transparent tentatively and briefly, and look for feedback from clients. How can I disclose something succinctly yet meaningfully, and then read cues from clients, particularly cues that what I have said is not helpful?

After any type of disclosure, keep turning the conversation back to clients' concerns and their story. What links can I make to what clients have already talked about?

Scan and make sure that you are in emotional control of what you are going to share. Where am I emotionally with what I am planning to talk about? Have I reflected enough on it to understand and present it from different angles?

Make sure that you are not expecting a particular reaction from clients following what you tell them. Be open to their experience but also prepared for them to reject what you say, make sure it is offered tentativily so that they can reject it comfortably if they need to. How I present something will convey an expectation with regard to what kind of reaction I anticipate unless I think about phrasing.

Offer information in a way that emphasises challenges you have faced rather than ideas of success/failure and solutions. Is this information likely to be of use to the client's thought processes?

Think about how presenting information from your life or about your theoretical beliefs or values will affect alliances within a family consultation of the PWA. In what ways are family members taking different sides with regard to different communication challenges? Do they differ in the way they see the PWA now? How might what I say affect therapeutic alliances or familial dynamics?

What are the spoken and unspoken rules in the work setting with regard to disclosure? What is already being communicated about your beliefs and life experience by being in that setting?

Create, share, and write treatment plans or reports with clients. How can you ensure that the ultimate ownership of the telling of their experience with aphasia is in the hands of clients? Can you write a discharge report in the form of a letter to your client, which is from an authentic version of yourself?

(Roberts 2005)

Clients often report the shedding of friends and colleagues following a brain injury; even those who were once close don't seem to maintain the friendship. This only adds further to the devastating loss of one's language and change to identity. The former pillars of support in life seem to crumble away, reinforcing a sense of shame and helplessness. This, too, is about the 'self' of the other person. People are afraid of incompetence, of losing face, of not finding **a** solution for the PWA, so they avoid. They are not avoiding the PWA; they are avoiding themselves.

Over recent years, I have extended these kinds of questions to other aspects of my work as an SLT. When it comes to clinically supervising students or working with colleagues around discussing research and having case discussions, application of similar self-questioning leads me to have a greater understanding of others' challenges, as well as offering them greater responsibility for developing continuing professional development that fits with their own backgrounds.

Case: Susie the SLT

I was born and grew up in a remote part of Tanzania in East Africa, one of four children with three brothers. Acquiring English and Swahili simultaneously, it was not until I was much older that I became conscious of the existence of two separate languages in my mind. Strange as it may seem, from my young child's viewpoint, it was just one 'way' of talking with one group of people and another way with the other. Swahili words integrated into our family conversations (because they seemed more accurate descriptors for our environment than our language which grew from an entirely different cultural context), but not vice versa. I spent many hours from being a baby until ten years of age with a young woman Maria who helped in the family with domestic tasks, but spoke no English. I remember being intrigued as a young child by the way her intonation, prolonged vowels, and facial expression conveyed meanings that were altogether 'separate' from the words. I absorbed conversations, between adults, among children and between the two, a fascination for discourse which remains with me.

For a variety of reasons, and although my language development was normal, stimulated by a creative, teaching mother, and play with my brothers, I felt silenced as soon as I was outside my family and without Maria. I loved to listen and watch but preferred to be invisible and not drawn into others' conversations. In fact, when I was spoken to, I froze, as if my cover had suddenly been blown. I felt unable to speak, not knowing where to start, although my mind was full of thoughts. The chasm between my thoughts on what was being said, and the utterances of others seemed insurmountable. At times no doubt I was perceived as being stubborn, awkward or even rude, but my experience was that it was none of these; only paralysis. It is not hard to see how this experience, which has characterised a large part of my life, is mirrored in my encounters with people with aphasia; and the enormous desire I experience to help them to bridge a similar chasm. Sudden acquired aphasia is a psychological trauma for the person experiencing it.

Awareness of this at a conscious level has become important to me, however, as there are two sides to this experience, one which is helpful and one which is entirely unhelpful and potentially damaging. The latter is one I continually have to guard against, where I inadvertently embrace or even enjoy the power of being the one who can talk, in the presence of the one who can't. I must ensure that my motives are wholly to support the PWA to come out of that impasse, and to listen more than talk. I must also recognise that my experience is not their experience – somewhat similar but different – and be curious about what those differences are for them.

Linguistic curiosity led me to study linguistics, French and Swahili at university, where I discovered the interesting historical, linguistic and semantic features of French too. There are words in Swahili that I still use today; the adjective 'kali' holds a variety of meanings, but is no less evocative for this. It can mean 'strong', 'fierce', 'bitter', 'spicy', 'extreme', but combined with its noun seems to convey the semantics more meaningfully for me than its English equivalent, regardless of context.

Studying Swahili was a challenge; despite already speaking the language from having acquired it aurally, I had no idea where the written word began and ended (roots and morphemes are added together) and therefore my written language was full of errors until I re-learned its grammar. The 18 noun classes were less of a challenge to me as I relied on what 'sounded' right when uttered aloud. I am aware that my linguistic background is what draws me into the psycholinguistic aspects of aphasia.

I saw Sir Jonathan Miller on TV asking a person with aphasia to name ordinary pictures and this instantly fascinated me. An intelligent, highly educated aged man could not name a pen. The idea that he knew what it was but could suddenly no longer say it was intriguing to me. The man could produce some phrases and greetings with no difficulty but looked utterly stumped by simple objects. What was going on?

I went to observe the highly esteemed clinical aphasiologist Eirian Jones working with a patient at my local hospital. This clinched the deal; I wanted to know more about this. Again, my own past and present experience of what I 'knew' being altogether different from what I could express was played out here. Eirian's tenacity with digging deep into the workings of language processing and her utter conviction that her patients were not 'cognitively' impaired, drew me in, with my linguistic knowledge, to the psycholinguistic model of aphasia therapy. This is a model which I use to this day and one that I refuse to consider as being out of vogue and only limited to an impairment model of therapy (see Chapter 2).

Working for 24 years as a specialist speech and language therapist, I gradually absorbed new research, integrated it with the old and subtly began to alter my focus with experience. I was feeling uncomfortable with the ways of working within the directives handed down in the medical model of care, and increasingly felt I was failing students, clinicans, PWA and their families, but didn't know why, or how to change it. My retrospective observation since altering the approach to my work is that health professionals can become 'institutionalised' and stuck in patterns of working and relating to each other and to patients and that these patterns become hard to shift.

The concept of the genogram and social graces (Hills 2012) in systemic training enabled me to view the multiple layers of context that have influenced my life, choices and behaviour and to understand gender and cultural differences that have affected me. Looking at layers of context in my life has led to an attempt to do so in the lives of others when they are dealing with difficulty. The broader context is everything and has helped me not only in work but in lots of aspects of life, to be more open to new ideas, look for change in my clients in a different way, and to be more forgiving of my own inability to change people's lives for them.

Realising how identity is developed in interactions with others, and that conversations change people, I have formed an alternative view of my identity to the unhelpful one I previously held: I have changed my posture from one of 'mobilisation' (wanting to change things) to one of tranquillity after many years (Griffith et al. 1990) and I strive to give others space to do this for themselves after a brain injury. Self-compassion can be acquired through looking carefully at the wider context of our own stories. Self-compassion leads to more authentic compassion for others, as we seek to be open to and understand their stories too. After all, we CHOOSE to hear, ignore or silence old stories and this is what shapes our personal identities (Roberts 2005).

Janine Roberts has worked in cross-cultural settings, as have I; this is what makes her work resonate with me. She raises ideas about women feeling heard; silent families, listening to others, speaking in 'one voice and polyphonic voices' where feelings and inner voices are heard. I consider such aspects of discourse now with my clients and their families. Roberts describes how unspoken things take on a growing presence – the elephant in the room grows bigger, which makes me reflect on what is unspoken because it physically can't be uttered, and what is chosen not be talked about and why. A person with aphasia has to grapple with a new identity, changing roles within family and relationships, and we as SLTs find ourselves addressing how these things are communicated or otherwise for the PWA.

I have learned that strong feelings about a family experiencing aphasia, together with a desire to protect or 'rescue' a client, sometimes relates to my personal experiences and I have to work hard to think about alternative stories and hold on to hypotheses more lightly.

Examining aspects of my own contexts enables me to be forgiving of things that have happened to me in my life, a greater sense of freedom to view aphasia therapy through a wider lens. This includes willingness to try new things out, explore other disciplines and bring them to bear in my work with people with aphasia. I am better able to deal with difficulty within aphasia therapy and within families affected by aphasia, as I try to examine the wider context and not to try to find a source of 'blame' or certain causes for problems.

There is an African proverb in the Nguni language, 'umuntu ngumuntu ngabantu', which means 'a person is a person through other people' (Kubow and Min 2016). Desmond Tutu visited my home when I was a child, and he expresses this African philosophy on being human; 'A person is not basically an independent, solitary entity. A person is human precisely in being enveloped in the community of other human beings, in being caught up in the bundle of life' (in Benghu 1996).

In her autobiographical account *Out of Africa*, Isak Dinesen (1937) wrote that 'All sorrows can be borne if we can put them into a story.' The sense of isolation that aphasia brings within our already individualistic society cannot be underestimated. Helping people with aphasia to put their sorrows into a story about themselves can bring acceptance and hope. A systemic approach to aphasia therapy helps us to view the person 'as a person through others' and create a community in which to envelope that person in order to help them, and ourselves, on the way to becoming the best we can be.

References

Bateson, G.(1972) *Steps to an Ecology of Mind*. Paladin.

Baum, S. (2011) Positioning theory and relational risk-taking: Connections when working with adults with learning disabilities and their families. *Context, Apr;114*. Association for Family Therapy and Systemic Practice.

Becvar, D. S. and Becvar, R. J. (1999) *Systems Theory and Family Therapy: A Primer*. Second edition. University Press of America.

Burnham, J. (2005) 'Relational reflexivity: A tool for creating therapeutic relationships'. In C. Flaskas, B. Mason and A. Perlesz (Eds), *The Space Between. Experience, Context and Process in the Therapeutic Relationship*. Routledge.

Burnham, J. (2013). 'Developments in social GGRRAAACCEEESSS: Visible-invisible, voiced-unvoiced'. In I.-B. Krause (Ed.), *Cultural Reflexivity*. Karnac.

Constantine, M. G. and Kwan, K.-L. K. (2003), Cross-cultural considerations of therapist self-disclosure. *J. Clin. Psychol.*, 59: 581–588.

Dallos, R. and Draper, R. (2010). *An Introduction to Family Therapy*. Open University Press.

De Shazer, S. (1985). *Keys to Solutions in Brief Therapy*. W. W. Norton.

Eger, E. (2020) *The Gift: 12 Lessons to Save Your Life*. Ebury Publishing.

Dinesen, I. (1937) *Out of Africa*. Putnam.

Fredman, G. (2007) Preparing ourselves for the therapeutic relationship: Revisiting 'Hypothesising revisited'. *Human Systems: The Journal of Systemic Consultation and Management*, 18: 44–59.

Gale, J. and Newfield, N. (1992) A conversation analysis of a solution focussed therapy session. *Journal of Marital & Family Therapy*, 18, 153–165.

Griffith, J. L., Griffith, M. E. and Slovik, L. S. (1990), Mind-body problems in family therapy: Contrasting first- and second-order cybernetics approaches. *Family Process*, 29: 13–28.

Hardy, K.V. and Laszloffy, T.A. (1995), The cultural genogram: Key to training culturally competent family therapists. *Journal of Marital and Family Therapy*, 21: 227–237.

Harré, R., & van Langenhove, L. (1999). 'The dynamics of social episodes'. In R. T. Harré and L. van Langenhove (Eds), *Positioning theory. Moral Contexts of Intentional Action* (pp. 1–13). Oxford: Blackwell.

Hedges, F. (2005) *An Introduction to Systemic Therapy with Individuals: A Social Constructionist Approach*. Palgrave Macmillan.

Hills, J. (2012) *Introduction to Systemic and Family Therapy: A User's Guide*. Palgrave Macmillan.

Hornstrup, C., Loehr-Petersen, J., Gjengedal Madsen, J., Johansen,T. and Vinther Jensen, A. (2012) *Developing Relational Leadership: Resources for Developing Reflexive Organizational Practices*. Taos Institute Publications.

Kubow, P. K., Min, M. (2016). The cultural contours of democracy: Indigenous epistemologies informing South African citizenship. *Democracy and Education*, 24(2), Article 5.

Roberts, J. (2005) Transparency and self-disclosure in family therapy: Dangers and possibilities. *Family Process*. March;44(1): 45–65.

Rock, D. (2008) SCARF: A brain-based model for collaborating with and influencing others. *NeuroLeadership Journal*, 1: 44–52.

Vygotsky, L. S. (1962). *Thought and Language*. MIT Press.

Watts-Jones, T. D. (2010), Location of self: Opening the door to dialogue on intersectionality in the therapy process. *Family Process*, 49: 405–420.

Watzlawick, P., Beavin-Bavelas, J. and Jackson, D. (1967). *Pragmatics of Human Communication: A Study of Interactional Patterns, Pathologies and Paradoxes*. W. W. Norton.

5 First encounters

In this chapter we will talk about the significance and potential pitfalls of first encounters with the PWA in the SLT clinical setting. Mention must be made first, however, of the systemic ideas around how we prepare ourselves to meet the people with whom we will form a therapeutic relationship. As we saw in Chapter 4, Fredman (2004) advocates overt consideration of the therapist's contexts and feelings in the session and before it. Clearly as therapists we aim to respect the people we meet through our work, but we must also be fully aware that we are part of the therapeutic system and try to make space for the person to feel competent in our encounters.

The first session is particularly important, as it sets the tone for how therapy will follow on. Fredman suggests some specific reflexive questions to consider before meeting a client/family, such as 'what might this person want me to most appreciate about them?'; 'what am I communicating nonverbally about my own feelings?'; 'how shall I ask questions that invite an atmosphere of respect, safety and collaboration?' (Fredman 2007). Consider carefully who will attend the first encounter along with the client. A friend? The family? the caregiver? Whoever attends will influence that encounter for the client in different ways, something we should prepare for in advance, at the same time as thinking about others in the person's life who are not in the session.

Many areas in the UK offer six weeks of Early Supported Discharge (ESD) from hospital, where a rehabilitation assistant visits the patient at home to carry out SLT or physio or TO exercises which have been directed by a qualified therapist. ESD is overseen by SLTs but is normally carried out by generic rehabilitation workers, bringing its own dilemmas, as discussed in Chapter 2. ESD will not be the focus of discussion here. Post-ESD, or where ESD is not

77

DOI: 10.4324/9781003178613-5

available, the traditional model of first encounters typically involves 1–4 of the following steps, or a variation of these:

1 Read referral
2 Take a case history
3 Language assessment
4 Background information questionnaire about the persons social, educational and professional background from next of kin
5 Set goals
6 Embark on therapy (1:1 or group)
7 Review
8 Discharge.

In many settings, the information we receive about a client who has suffered a brain injury is determined by the content of the form that is completed by the referrer. A referral letter may give the medical diagnosis, e.g., haemorrhagic or ischaemic stroke with the site of lesion, the next of kin, and a brief medical history. The case history at the end of this chapter illustrates the need for caution when reading a referral letter about a PWA.

Sometimes we consider a referral to be 'inappropriate', and return it to the referring agency, when it turns out that the information reflected an inaccurate understanding of the condition. Case history proforma are often used in the initial session, for the purposes of uniformity and to ensure key points are not missed. The answers are reflected by the questions. They provide a form of scaffolding onto which to develop our work with the client. This means we worry less about omissions, because 'we have done what is required' on the form. This applies also to language assessments used; if we use a standardised measure of auditory sentence comprehension for example (e.g., Comprehensive Aphasia Test), this will tell us what kinds of lexical and grammatical structures presented have been understood in that particular task, and in the context of the clinic.

How many aphasia therapists later discard some of these forms because they fail to adequately represent the person that is in front of us? Language is a creative and unwieldy entity. Assessments and forms which try to capture it can act more like straitjackets than true depictions of a person's language.

The general public do not understand aphasia. GPs do not understand aphasia. Hospitals do not understand aphasia. Many SLTs do not truly understand aphasia (just as I as an SLT do not truly understand autistic spectrum disorder, paediatric dysphagia or numerous other areas in which SLTs work). These are facts. One 60-year-old single man I knew was assessed in hospital by a well-meaning social worker, in relation to where he was to be discharged to. His speech was jargonistic and his language comprehension very poor. In addition, he had little insight into this. His indication of a town on a map led to him being transported to a nursing home there. It was only when he was seen by an SLT some months later that it transpired he had been showing the social worker where he was born, not where he now lived and wanted to continue living, close to family and friends. It took several months to move him back to where he should have been in the first place. Of course, there is no reason why the social worker should fully understand aphasia; not all stroke patients have aphasia. However, the presence of an SLT could have prevented this misunderstanding and the ensuing distress it caused. Unfortunately, however, it is often the case that PWA and their families are offered inaccurate, assumptive predictions about recovery from aphasia, from people who hold the powerful positions of trust that we discussed in the last chapter. When this happens, the PWA is robbed of hope, which is the most precious resource they/we have.

Aphasia groups on social media (e.g., Aphasia Recovery, Talk Aphasia) abound with stories of being told 'you will not improve after 6 months', 'you have reached a plateau of recovery', 'why don't you take up horse riding', all by medical professionals, and the devastating consequences of such predictions. A gentleman referred very recently to me from a London hospital was told by his neurologist that he must take up speech therapy now because if he didn't, it would be too late to change, as he would have reached six months (most of that during lockdown). I wonder what experience this neurologist has of talking to people with aphasia he has treated, two years, five years and eleven years from seeing them? Sadly, this is not an unusual story.

I have seen people whose aphasia remained unchanged for six months before even starting to change. It is not too extreme to say that the linguistic power held over the person with aphasia in the medical setting silences them and disempowers their families. They are faced, then, with not only getting over the practical consequences of having aphasia but also the consequences of this advice on their mental health.

Derek moved to my local area two years after his stroke. His new GP referred him for his mild-moderate expressive aphasia, stipulating in his referral letter that he knew 'it is very unlikely you will be able to help him at this stage'.

(Had he also given this awful news to the man himself, I wondered?) Derek's wife was very worried as he seemed to be in a deep depression, despite a fresh start locally.

Derek was prescribed antidepressants from his GP but continued to feel 'empty' and 'hopeless'. I was interested as to why Derek and his wife had not sought SLT until now, so I asked him about his hospital stay at the time of his stroke. He told me:

> 'The consultant said it would take two years to get my speech back and that speech therapy doesn't really make a difference, it will get better of its own accord. It is now 2 years and 2 months, and my speech is still not back to normal. I'm still fitting kitchens rather than doing the sales work I used to do, and I can't take the waiting anymore.'

Derek's understanding of what was said to him led him to wait for two years, expecting change to happen. Nobody in this time checked his understanding of this with him or challenged the advice. (SLTs are aware that, even if a PWA appears to be understanding what is said to them, particularly in the acute phase of treatment, information processing is often impaired which affects comprehension.) Regardless of whether Derek had processed or retained this information accurately, this is what he took away with him and it prevented him and his wife from seeking support and treatment until things had become intolerable for him.

It is important to be aware of the limitations of our knowledge. I would not dream of advising a parent about her infant's dysphagia (and not only because she is capable of questioning my knowledge). I do not wish to give her anything that will undermine her ability to get through this difficulty, impacting on her infant's or her own mental health. Instead, I will listen, acknowledge and be transparent about my ignorance and refer her to a colleague that knows and understands and can show her where hope lies. My role with Derek became about exploring and reframing his understanding and experience of aphasia to date in a way that he could begin to move forward with his life.

We discover that every PWA and the context they live in is unique. We interact with each and every client in a unique manner, but as SLTs I would suggest we struggle to articulate how we do this, and we struggle to feel that what we are offering is truly meaningful and helpful to the client and their families. At this point, in the life of the recently qualified SLT, dysphagia,

LSVT, dysarthria and other intra-SLT subjects start to become far more attractive as clinical areas in which they can make a tangible difference, whilst remaining emotionally distanced. For me, it is not enough to merely accept the polite gratitude of clients who often thank us so generously for seeing them, I want to know how to ensure they have ongoing hope.

Caregivers

The word caregiver here refers to a 'close other' of the PWA, whomever that may be. The experience of many caregivers of a loved one with a neurological injury has been that whilst medical care addresses the body of the PWA, neurologists and doctors can communicate in an unkind, unsympathetic manner, devoid of humanistic awareness of the devastation of this extraordinary life event. One lady told me that a neurologist stood by her husband's bedside and told her that this was the end of treatment, 'Just make him comfortable at home, he won't walk or talk again but you can give him his PEG feeds and hold his hand. I will discharge him tomorrow.' What was most distressing for her was the real possibility that her husband also heard the neurologist appear to give up hope for him.

A caregiver becomes an advocate for the patient with aphasia whilst in hospital. Relatives tell me that where conversation is almost impossible, physical touch becomes a lifeline of communication; it reassures the PWA when the fear of suddenly discovering they cannot communicate is overwhelming.

For some, the fear of being abandoned by loved ones is very real. Carers must deal with the physical and financial burden of caring. Some PWA are of working age; the minefields of disability benefits, looking after children, elderly parents, all fall on the caregiver. They are coping with their own shock, grief and loss, and are also on the receiving end of tremendous grief and loss experienced by the PWA. On top of this, the PWA and their caregiver struggle to communicate with aphasia. If they are having drop-in carers at home, they have yet another job of training the carer in how to communicate with their loved ones as they are being washed, dressed, etc. Some caregivers do abandon their partners on discharge, some committing suicide, so overwhelmed are they by the prospect of the future. I have been in the position more than once, of telling a person with severe aphasia that their partner is not able to be their carer and will be moving away from them.

It is a normal part of grieving for caregivers to initially refuse to accept what has happened, because they don't want to have such upheaval in their life. Ambiguous loss occurs when the person is still present but not in the same way as before and can be accompanied by overwhelming feelings of guilt. The PWA might feel helpless and childlike but know their intellect is intact. The caregiver may crack, treating the PWA like a child even when they know they aren't. It is all part of the tangled web of relationality. Perhaps this is the point at which we meet them in our clinic? Is it any wonder they feel angry and exhausted, when they are feeling their partner's pain as well as their own?

One spouse told me that whilst they felt abandoned by the medical world, the SLT, OT and physiotherapists gave him his wife back over the three years following her stroke. He often felt lonely, at times he needed to explode, go outside and scream and shout, his feelings of anger were frequent, and sometimes he shouted at his wife, or she would throw something at him. Feelings of guilt and sadness followed.

Caregivers also need to be heard and supported, in hospital and in the community, so that PWA are protected, and the caregivers' experiences of distress normalised. It is ok to ask the caregiver in that first meeting: 'What is going on at the moment emotionally for you both', 'How are you getting on with caring for each other?'

There are times when SLTs encounter clients or family members who are angry and express hostility towards the therapist. I was often forewarned about clients and families who are 'angry' and 'verbally abusive' as somebody in the office may well have already received an irate telephone call and shared hits with the therapist.

People often feel freer to express strong feelings over the phone to a faceless entity that to them represents the health system that they feel powerless against. I used to 'prepare my defence' prior to meeting such clients. It is natural to want to defend our positions. Overwhelmed by busy caseloads, training and administrative demands of the job and by our clients' grief, there is a certain amount of 'self-preservation' that takes place so that we can still function within our own family and work positions. As the speech and language therapist, we are often the only outsiders who sit with the family to hear their stories about communication breakdown and the associated distress. I am not sure how well we prepare our students for this.

Prior to taking on systemic training, when I already had many years' experience behind me, I began to be more interested in those 'difficult' clients following a particularly memorable event. I recall sitting before the extremely angry wife of a person with moderate aphasia on a gloomy winter's day in February. One of my own children was ill, I was sleep-deprived, exhausted and singularly unmotivated for the day's work ahead of me. A petite, well-dressed woman furiously thrust her husband (who had also lost much of his mobility) into my room in his wheelchair.

She made no eye contact with me at all but launched into a tirade peppered with expletives about how they had been appallingly treated, that the hospital in Derby where he was treated was excellent, she should have stayed there as they did everything for him. She banged her hand down on the table violently with almost every syllable and my headache ricocheted in my skull with each strike. Since returning to their home on a mobile home site, she said, they had been abandoned and nobody was doing anything. She supposed I wouldn't do anything either as I was 'probably just useless as the rest of them in this ******* hellhole of a county'. 'He just sits there saying nothing and doesn't even try to help, I have to do everything, he is useless – tell me, you ****ing expert, tell me what I should do.' I looked with alarm at the blank emotionless expression on her husband's face as she shoved his shoulder aggressively.

Such was my own feeling of helplessness and despair in that moment, that I immediately abandoned my usual 'script' for people who come seeking information and help with aphasia.

I was faced with the choice of either asking them to leave until she had calmed down, or deal with it, and I didn't know how to. I felt defensive of him and of myself; safeguarding thoughts floated by, and I felt threatened by her behaviour; I was about to prove to her what she was telling me – how useless I would be. Feeling my head was about to burst, I just sat and waited until she ran out of steam momentarily. I asked her by name to stop talking, to look at me and to sit down and tell me all about it more slowly, step by step. I said I needed her to stop swearing so that I could understand what was happening for her (and protect my head!) and listen to the words that mattered.

This woman was from a very different social world to my own. Behind her words I heard she felt alone and frightened and had previously depended on her husband to make all the decisions about their lives. In spite of the 'amazing treatment' in Derby, it transpired that she was referring to the acute care, when he was being treated and she wasn't having to care for him. In fact, she had never heard of the word 'aphasia', she said, and thought that he was just refusing to speak to be awkward. It is very likely she was told he had aphasia, but this woman was in such a heightened state of distress that she was struggling to process any information beyond her immediate survival needs. Listening to her story, acknowledging her anger and validating her concerns transformed the session from bedlam into a constructive plan for intervention.

An ecological approach

I later came to realise that by being forced to let go of the 'knowledge' and the power that we hold up to our clients, I could be interested in the reasons for their distress, or their dissatisfaction, and I began to listen more actively. I began to see anger as an expression of fear and a request for help. I learned that some clients who are very amenable and agree with you may be doing so because you have the power and just find it hard to disagree with you, even if what you advise doesn't fit their lives. Anderson and Goolishian (1992) advise that in family therapy we should not be afraid of what we might hear, as it is only when you get it all out that you can start the work of co-construction, a more helpful way of being.

Systemic training taught me a great deal more about the impact of aphasia on clients and families from different narrative backgrounds. More importantly, these are the clients with whom, together, we ultimately reached the most successful outcomes that were not related to their score on a language test.

The neurosurgeon Paul Kalanithi talks about his own learning through the experience of being a patient:

> Openness to human relationality does not mean revealing grand truths from the apse it means meeting patients where they are, in the narthex or nave and bringing them as far as you can. A physician's duty is to take into our arms a patient and family whose lives have disintegrated and work until they can stand back up and face and make sense of their own existence.

He explains that his doctor did not give him back his old identity, but 'she protected my ability to forge a new one' (Kalanithi 2016) I think our role as SLTs is not so far from this when it comes to the person with aphasia and their loved ones.

Aphasia therapists often remark on the hard work and practice that PWA and their caregivers are willing to put into their recovery. If communication is what makes us human, we will fight to retain and develop our communication in order to stay part of the communities and families on whom we depend for our survival.

In order to find out how well the person understands conversations that happen in the family, or if and how and when they participate at work or in their community, we need to ask different questions and talk to different people. I learned through systemic training to ask questions I thought I knew the answer to. Experimenting with this, I was surprised to find that the answer was different from the one I expected. I was not understanding as well as I thought.

The kinds of questions we ask, and how we ask them, will determine what and how therapy proceeds. As we saw in Chapter 4, the questions we ask are influenced by our own personal stories. Presenting our clients with forms and paperwork establishes our position in relation to them; we are in control and we are capturing their predicament on these sheets of paper, in order to advise them on how to step forward with aphasia. I am not suggesting that paperwork serves no use. However, I fervently believe that if we adopt a more ecological approach to working with people with aphasia then we can maintain our professional stance in a way that is more meaningful to the client and can be extended into the contexts of their families, work and friends.

A 'more ecological approach' forms the basis of a systemic approach to therapy. It asks questions such as 'What meaning do I take from this referral information?', 'What is it not telling me?', 'How do I present a language assessment in a way that does not feel threatening? What is the client thinking, what is the partner thinking and what does it mean for the language tasks, and the work of aphasia therapy?'

There is already the job to be done in creating a hypothesis around the aphasia impairment, but it is also about being curious about what is important for the client in the context of their lives, and how talking about this in different ways might open up change for the client. It is about how we create, with the client, a new context for our work, where we interact mutually into the contexts of each other's lives.

Circular questioning already discussed in this book helps us to explore the experience of a difficulty for a client and the context in which they operate. Circular questioning skills emanate from the Milan systemic approach to family therapy (Tomm 1985), as a means of navigating a problem that a client brings. This is done 'naively' with the client, so the therapist doesn't have the answers, the client doesn't yet know they have the answers, but it places the evolving expertise firmly in the hands of the client. In aphasia therapy, such questions can shed light on connections (e.g., what is it about my interactions with my partner that are changed because of aphasia?) and distinctions (e.g., when it is quiet I can find my words more easily). Of course, we can tell the PWA that they will find it easier when it is quiet, but will they not derive more meaning from this if they identify this themselves as being true, through their own experience?

Asking a question tentatively, which may be part of an initial hypothesis, stimulates a response, and this 'live' feedback is used to formulate the next question, and so on, thus adapting one's hypothesis continually until the client feels that what is being said is true for their experience. Skillful use of circular questioning can help to gain an understanding of others' perspectives on the aphasia, both for the therapist and the client. Of particular significance is that the client can begin to use their own self-knowledge and resource to identify answers to the questions posed that they didn't know they had.

Referrals to a speech and language therapist for aphasia therapy unwittingly 'tell a story' about a client. Factual medical information is included but will often include a description of the problem as understood by the referrer e.g., 'speech difficulty', 'understands everything but can't talk', 'wife very anxious' or 'family unhappy with service they have received'. Such descriptions can be 'totalising' and can prejudice the perspective of the receiving therapist before the client has even entered the room. Definitive statements can leave little room for alternative, and perhaps more lifelike descriptions which allow for variability, change, and most importantly hope. The difference to the therapy we offer depends on how we respond to that information. Many SLTs will testify to being very surprised when they meet someone whose referral information appears to belong to a different person, when they finally meet face to face.

One of the most significant things I have learned is that when meeting someone for the first time I must put to one side my own 'knowledge' about health, hospitalisation, brain injury and processes in healthcare, so I can meet that person where they are at that moment in time. We forget how immersed we are in the systems in which we work, how alien this might be to the PWA and their family, and this distances us from the client; it forms part of the power dynamic and prevents us from truly hearing what the client has to say. We forget how the client might view us from their position but by thinking differently we can learn to be mindful of this.

If we focus from the outset on treatment alone, what we are telling the client is that we expect to offer remediating therapy. Why are we surprised, when further down the line we struggle with discharging clients from the caseload? (This will be discussed in Chapter 7).

Our healthcare system offers a world of difference between the hospital-based acute phase of care and the availability of community-based rehabilitation. Clinicians often (not always, admittedly) work in either one setting or the other, which means they do not understand either what the client is coming from, or going to, depending on their own location.

Relationship to help

Explanations about aphasia are given in hospital, where the person is passively being cared for; relatives may visit and want prognostic information from medical staff and therapists. No matter how accurate (and I would argue it is almost impossible to be accurate at this stage) the information given, people reassess that information in the light of returning home to where they start to become aware of the enormity of that change that has taken place. Often, they will refute they had ever been told anything; processing such life-changing information is a huge challenge in the acute setting. Hospital staff may be unaware of what provision is available to the PWA, beyond the six-week ESD programme, and how large a chasm the patient and their family are about to fall into.

Experiencing a stroke or other cause for brain injury and the experience of hospitalisation for most people is new and frightening. People come to therapy with great uncertainty about what their brain injury all means. As medical professionals, for whom the medical setting provides us with our livelihood, colleagues, friends and a sense of 'safety', we 'forget' to see things from the perspective of a patient for whom autonomy has evaporated and who believe that their impairment is the only thing of interest to the clinician.

We all have our own 'relationship to help' (Burnham 2005; Reder and Fredman 1996), including us therapists. For some people, being helped is an intolerable situation to be in; they may view themselves as the person who helps others, for example. Accepting help for some people is experienced as disempowering and highly distressing. For others, being helped is so much part of their experience that self-management may be a real challenge.

Just as hypothesis testing is intrinsic to aphasiology, so should we apply this approach to trying to understand the context of the person with aphasia and their close others, including their relationship to help, for example. We might want to know more about how aphasia has affected the family as well as how the family has affected the aphasia; in other words, how the family system manages change in general, what arises as a result of the aphasia and how members respond.

PWA aphasia often seem to expect or want a statement as to what to do about the aphasia. In systemic approaches, therapists set a context for change to have the most chance of taking place. For the SLT it is difficult not to give a statement at the outset as to what the client or family must do, but PWA and their families live within a unique set of contexts and a unique family 'story'. The 'script' by which they live their lives may be very different from our own and we should be open to that.

It takes time and the careful development of a therapeutic relationship in order to share the balance of power. In my experience conversations really need to start with what the person understands about what has happened to them.

Community SLT

In the UK community SLT services are insufficient to cater for the number of people with aphasia requiring speech and language therapy. As previously mentioned, waiting lists are normally held. People with aphasia and their families become very anxious when waiting for an appointment, especially when they are aware of the media information to act fast with a stroke and get help as soon as possible. The news that the waiting time may be several months, if the service is available at all, results in confusion, helplessness and greater sense of loss and shame. Waiting times, set at 12 weeks, take a linear approach, based on the NHS resources available, not on what is clinically most useful for individuals. Services may also stipulate how many sessions a client can receive, when they do reach the top of the list.

In my community NHS post, I found that if I arranged to see the referred PWA as soon as possible after discharge from hospital, rather than rely on the perspective of the referrer, I would be far better informed as to how to triage them (in relation to other referrals). In addition, I could already start some of the work with them in that first appointment. This approach had two outcomes.

First, this helped me with the practical task of managing the waiting list; once the person had been really heard, discussed their fears and concerns, and received an explanation about what had happened, what may or may not happen in the future, in a way they could understand, and been reassured there was support available when they needed it, I was surprised to find that they became less 'needy' and more autonomous around their therapy. It is interesting to consider here, whether this approach also made me as a therapist, less 'needy' of the desire to be the exclusive solver of problems for that person! They seemed to feel that they had some control over their recovery, and perhaps very importantly they could ask to see the therapist on their own terms. Far from inundating me with requests, particularly about how soon and how often they can be seen, therapy sessions and phone calls were productive and useful for both therapist and client. They had not waited for weeks, becoming more and more anxious and 'helpless', convinced of some 'magic answer' that they were being deprived of by being on a waiting list.

Second, people often came back to seek therapy later on at their own stage of readiness; the work was already on the way to being done, they had begun to learn about their strengths and difficulties and about their loved one's strengths and difficulties in being able to support them. Acknowledging the difficulty of conversations with newly acquired aphasia and identifying some ways with which to approach these without criticism and self-blame, led to the emergence of further resources that were already owned by the client and their family.

I was fortunate enough to have a manager who understood aphasia and allowed me clinical freedom. We offered open access to therapy so that people with aphasia could return to the service at any time. They were not limited to a certain number of sessions. Such an approach is entirely in keeping with the Department of Health's National Stroke Strategy guidelines (2007) which advocate availability of help for survivors of stroke *when they need it*. The guidelines' quality marker 3 advises that 'People who have had a stroke, and their relatives and carers, have access to practical advice, emotional support, advocacy and information throughout the care pathway and lifelong.'

Just as in systemic family therapy, I have found that often the work takes place outside and between sessions; the clinical session is where the seeds of that progress might be sown but the person's rehabilitation is not dependent only on the time spent with you alone. Understanding this is key to enabling therapists to demonstrate their competence, being more open to trying different approaches and ready to discard what doesn't work; realising that the client may find it hard to disagree with you but creating the opportunity for them to do so safely. All this has a surprisingly positive effect on the therapeutic relationship. Systemic therapists would say that positive connotation in this way considers differences in power. It also helps people to progress, as the client is the expert (Anderson and Goolishian 1992).

I found that among any PWA referred for SLT, severity of the aphasia does not correlate with either the amount of therapy they require or the ability to cope with the change that it brings to their life. A linear, medical view assumes that a person described as having severe aphasia will be wanting numerous sessions over long periods of time, so the tendency in a busy clinic is to allocate less time for those with 'mild' aphasia. Some of the most distressed people I have worked with are those with relatively mild impairment who struggle to imagine that a future without the full language function they previously owned is possible. In fact, I have often found that higher functioning patients take longer, as you spend much more time dealing with adjustment processes and family adjustment. Other factors, such as living alone, personality, the nature of their close relationships, their interests, are more likely to influence the level of support needed but these are hard to quantify.

A person who suffers huge changes in physical, communication, and cognitive functioning as a result of brain injury, will undergo change in almost every aspect of their life, as may their caregiver. Life can be entirely altered, and it is clearer what has to happen. For those who experience just aphasia, say, even mild aphasia, the process of coming to terms with what is, for them, ambiguous loss also, can be more problematic.

John was a businessman whose sons and wife took over the running of the business immediately following a stroke which left him with only very mild aphasia after six weeks. Feeling confident that this would continue to improve, I was surprised how depressed and lacking confidence he seemed. He felt 'redundant' now, his sons ran the business, his wife did the books, and everyone kept him away, telling him not to worry, protecting him from stress. I suggested he might exercise to increase his breath support for his speech, raise endorphins to enhance his mood, and benefit from the protective cardiovascular gains. He loved swimming, but his wife was too embarrassed to go swimming unless he built a pool in their garden. When I suggested he approach his local baths to ask for a supervised session, his response was 'If I went swimming alone, it would be like a kick in the face to my wife'. He was 'allowed' to invite a neighbour to come and play table tennis. His wife insisted he wait for her to go for a walk, even though she had a leg injury which meant he could only walk with her at a very slow pace.

On closer discussion, I learned that she worries about him having another stroke so much that he will not do things without her approval in case it causes her more worry. He volunteered, 'I think we prevent each other from doing things by mistake, because we don't want to upset each other. I asked whether waiting for permission to do things or having to weigh up his choices in case they cause worry may be contributing to his feeling of being 'redundant'. He said he thought we had hit the nail on the head. He also said she has some serious health issues which worry her and so he doesn't want to add to this. I wondered aloud how she would feel if he started making his own choices and doing things for himself; could this actually reduce the load she feels? He may be inadvertently reinforcing her worry. We then talked about how he could reassure his wife that he could swim while she is at work and then go for a slow walk with her later, and that there are lifeguards and he will build up gradually and stop if he feels unwell; he is being sensible. I found that really listening to him and trying to understand the context for his depression, listening to his choice of words and turns of phrase, allowed me to ask him to explain further and he then came up with a practical solution for making a change.

Normally I would have made suggestions and reassured him about his speech, without appreciating how the dynamics of his relationship were causing the depression that his wife told me she was concerned about and that he denied, although he did not deny feeling redundant, and doing nothing. I feel that if he can regain some control of his life, both parties will benefit and their relationship will improve so they can enjoy things more, and he has more things to talk about.

We can protect others so much that we handicap them. John was in a position of trying to please his family by complying with their wishes; unsurprisingly he became very depressed as a result. 'I should feel grateful to them for helping me, if I do it without them, they think I don't need them, and they get upset. The last thing I want to do is upset them.' Here is an example of a dilemma which is less about aphasia and more about family scripts, relationships to help and helping.

A joint session with John and his wife resulted in the couple discussing these issues openly with one another in the therapy session: the session became therapeutic, even though the focus was not aphasia. John was worried his wife was making herself ill running the business and wanted her to hand it over to their sons, both of whom were living with them, together with partners, in order to save up for mortgages. John's wife coped with difficulty by immersing herself in activity and being in control.

Can we really draw a line between aphasia therapy and family therapy or is there a case for a combined, i.e., systemic approach in supporting families with aphasia? Harlene Anderson exhorts therapists to 'Always be the learner, the client a teacher' when working with families (Anderson 2001). In her view, if you give clients your undivided attention, they will find their way. I have found this also to be true in my work. I have come to believe, like the Milan therapists, that solutions to dilemmas are often to be found within the individual or family. I find that these solutions are the ones that work out best; this relates to the key systemic idea that if the client has a sense of having drawn on their own resources and knowledge, it increases the possibility they will look to themselves to deal with future challenges (Hills 2012). If we can help the PWA to deal with the future challenges of aphasia long after our interventions have ended, we are on the way to having done our job.

Having heard as much as I can of the PWA's experience so far, I will then draw a very simplistic, visual explanation of lateralisation first of all (see Fig.5.1a). Gradually, I will add to the sketch the location of neurological damage and the ways which this affects language processing, all the time pointing out the vast areas of preserved function in the brain (Fig.5.1 b). The final additions to the sketch show how neuroplasticity can occur and how 'a diversion can develop with increased efficiency around the obstruction' (Fig. 5.1c). This also helps to explain how 'comprehension' difficulties can be seen in terms of inefficient information processing rather than simply not being able to understand. Using a visual model such as this, however crude, offers the PWA the chance to request clarification, ask questions, express confusion and so on.

I check for acknowledgement by the person that they actually experience, say, knowing the word but being unable to say it, validating their experience of having the word ready and then it disappearing from their grasp, knowing what someone has said to them but not really fully registering its meaning.

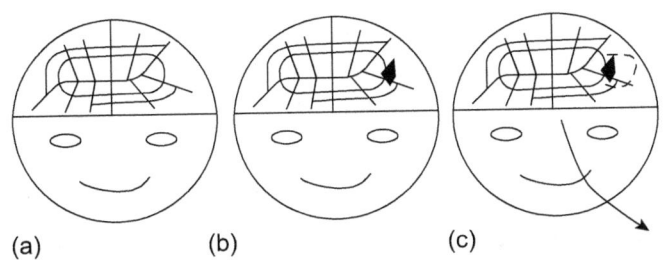

Figure 5.1 Supported conversation sketch of aphasia

The complete and utter exhaustion of neurological fatigue. This process is part of the PWA feeling heard.

I do not need to tell qualified SLTs how to do a language assessment in this book. Language assessment carried out on the background described in this chapter will be far more meaningful for client and therapist, and far more likely to foster engagement, as a sound therapeutic relationship and trust can begin to form.

Personally, I do not view assessment as being separate from therapy; rather assessment and therapy are intertwined from the outset; 'diagnostic' therapy is an ongoing process and therapy is a dynamic process which must adapt and move with the client. Collecting background information from the family about the PWA is better done at this stage, rather than prior to meeting them, as the family will now begin to understand why they are being asked for this, have confidence that it will be used sensitively, and the questions can be tailored to fit what the therapist has heard already about the person's priorities and hopes. Alternatively, it may form part of the goal-setting process, which will be discussed in Chapter 6.

Case: Magda

Magda was 15 when a hit and run driver left her with a severe traumatic brain injury. She was a bright student who had wanted to become a nurse or a physiotherapist. She lived with her Polish-speaking mother and younger siblings in a run-down area of town, where there was significant alcohol and drug misuse, burglary and assaults. Her father had returned to Poland after losing his job prior to her accident.

Magda was being seen periodically by a paediatric MDT following her discharge from hospital. She had returned home with considerable communication and cognitive difficulties. Living at a considerable distance from the brain injury service, Magda had no means of travel from her home; therefore, professional input was minimal at this stage. Added to this, her mother understood very little English; Magda had been the main interpreter for the family, having been at school in the country since the age of 6, and now she struggled to talk.

My involvement came when Magda was turning 18, as I specialise in working with adults. I struggled to understand the complex nature of her rehabilitation story, such as it was. I was surprised to hear that she was attending a college for young people with learning disability. She had virtually 1:1 supervision at all times, whilst her old friends had moved on to sixth form colleges. Her educational sessions included learning to read and write on a developmental programme, carried out by staff who were familiar with working with learning disability. She kept absconding and there were concerns about her safety in the local community, given that she had some memory difficulties. Magda, it turned out, was very skilled at masking her marked communication difficulty. (Probably because she did not have a learning disability!) Referrals had been made to the adult SLT service locally; however they declined to see Magda as they 'do not provide an SLT service for adults with learning disability'. All clinicians I spoke to involved with Magda expressed frustration, concern and helplessness over this particular case, as nobody had any solutions as to where to go next, and they were worried for her future.

A lack of availability of services locally is hard to overcome. However, by taking a holistic view of Magda's situation it was possible to identify the type of support that was likely to be most useful to this young woman.

I started by talking to all clinical professionals involved in her case, her social worker, her teachers and her local Headway service. I obtained a linear account of what had taken place in chronological order.

Assessment reports by the MDT contained 'problem-saturated' accounts of Magda's presentation in the early stages of her recovery. Some of her difficulties had in fact resolved but were still being referred to as being current aspects of her presentation. Indeed, some remarks were interpreted as being diagnostic when they were not intended to be so!

For example, an early psychological assessment showed Magda's performance on a task to be 'within the range of an adult with a learning disability'. This wording, together with her young age and being in fulltime education, ultimately led to the decision by those looking through the lens of her 'educational needs' (i.e., reading and writing ability as measured by developmental norms) to categorise her as being a student with a learning disability. This environment was one where all the young adults had a developmental physical and/or learning disability and had all attended special schools locally. Teachers were trained in special education, and not brain injury.

Then I met Magda.

What I had read bore little relationship to the client in front of me. Magda was physically well, and she used to like to swim regularly. She had a warm, loving family at home, greatly concerned for her welfare and willing to transcend language barriers by whatever means possible. Friendly, with an engaging communication style, Magda was polite and pleasant to interact with. Her social communication was good, she initiated exchanges and was very communicative through her facial expressions. When she wasn't understood by others, she was quick to try gestures, and she was adept at navigating her phone and iPad, within the limits of her language processing ability.

Magda came across as very motivated to improve and get on with life, she engaged with SLT sessions and reported finally feeling understood – 'at last, someone gets it!' She was clearly working hard to process my questions, greatly helped by written key words and checking in on her understanding as we went along. She expressed frustration when trying to respond, and teared up when I asked her whether she 'knew' the words in her head but couldn't access them.

There had been no mention of aphasia in her assessments. However, SLT assessment using the Comprehensive Aphasia Test and aspects of the PALPA revealed Magda's overriding impairment to be aphasia. (Mild cognitive communication factors such as fatigue and memory were so secondary to this significant communication disability, aphasia had not been addressed and therefore Magda had not been 'heard', so I decided aphasia would be targeted in therapy straight away.)

Cuespeak, an app devised by Jon Hunt, provides a comprehensive resource for assessing as well as treating psycholinguistic functioning in a topical, context-bound and intuitive manner. It aims to recreate real-life interactions, and regularly updates with topical issues that have been in the news, making it feel relevant to younger people. Magda found she could retrieve the words with the help of some context and semantic cues; she could spell simple words and recognise when she got them right; she smiled at the 'results' of each task, taking up the challenge to demonstrate her competence, not only at word-finding with support, but also with her ability to operate and navigate the app independently. This helped to confirm for me that her overwhelming difficulty was in fact aphasia, and, more importantly, that I could offer her some therapy that would effectively target her underlying impairment.

Additional interventions focussed on training college and Headway staff about aphasia. Systemically, Magda and I presented her story as one of strengths as well as difficulties, helping to alter the narrative of those around her as well as her own narrative to one of inherent competence. Although a formal SLT report with assessment results etc. was also provided, it was important for the entire team to receive the same information and therefore it had to be accessible by all involved to ensure maximum communication around supporting the client. For this I used the Aphasia Etiquette YouTube link, which is designed for doctors but easily understood by lay people, removing much of the 'mystery' that surrounds aphasia.

Magda started to attend a Headway service part-time, which immediately began to address her independent living skills with a skilled neuro occupational therapist and provide a supportive social environment in which she could be supported to communicate. She could demonstrate her competence in cooking, socialising, woodwork, using computers and handling money.

Developing skills of supported conversation in the people who surround the person with aphasia is crucial. Information on aphasia in Polish was provided to the family, with links to aphasia websites for further support and information.

Finally, working with the adult SLT service, I explained that she did not in fact have a diagnosis of learning disability and she was duly placed on their waiting list for outpatient therapy. This was to be delivered by a remotely supervised band 5 (newly qualified) therapist as the service in the area was so stretched.

Coming from outside the 'system' that was involved in Magda's care, it was possible to widen the lens beyond the scripts of the organisations which had responsibility for her and which worked to their own professional mores e.g., learning disability, education, medical care, social services, the family and so on.

References

Anderson, H. (2001) Postmodern and collaborative and person-centred therapies: What would Carl Rogers say? *Journal of Family Therapy*, 23(4): 339–361.

Anderson, H. and Goolishian, H. (1992) 'The client is the expert: A not-knowing approach to therapy'. In S. McNamee and K. J. Gergen (Eds), *Therapy as Social Construction* (pp. 25–39). Sage.

Burnham, J. (2005) 'Relational reflexivity: A tool for socially constructing therapeutic relationships'. In C. Flaskas, B. Mason, A. Perlesz (Eds), *The Space Between. Experience, Context, and Process in the Therapeutic Relationship*. Routledge.

Fredman, G. (2004) *Transforming Emotion: Conversations in Counselling and Psychotherapy*. John Wiley & Sons.

Fredman, G. (2007) Preparing ourselves for the therapeutic relationship. Revisiting 'Hypothesis revisited'. *Human Systems: The Journal of Systemic Consultation and Management*, 18: 44–59.

Hills, J. (2012) *Introduction to Systemic and Family Therapy: A User's Guide*. Palgrave Macmillan.

Kalanithi, P. (2016) *When Breath Becomes Air*. Random House.

National Stroke Strategy (2007) Department of Health, UK. Available at: https://nsnf.org.uk/assets/documents/dh_081059.pdf

Reder, P. and Fredman, G. (1996) The relationship to help: Interacting beliefs about the treatment process. *Clinical Child Psychology and Psychiatry*, 1(3): 457–467.

Tomm, K. (1985) 'Circular interviewing: A multifaceted clinical tool'. In D. Campbell and R. Draper (Eds), *Applications of Systemic Family Therapy*. Academic Press.

6 | Reaching for goals

Goal setting

Goal setting is considered to be an essential part of providing focused, time-sensitive rehabilitation. Many people believe it is the best way to structure rehabilitation and ensures one is dealing with clinically relevant problems (Wilson et al. 2009, Royal College of Physicians 2012).

Good rehabilitation should set meaningful, challenging but achievable goals, according to Wade (1999). Worrall et al. (2011) relate goals to the International Classification of Functioning, Disability and Health (ICF) classification approved by the World Health Organisation. They refer to findings that suggest that identifying the goals of individuals in rehabilitation allows meaningful and effective intervention to take place (McPherson and Siegert, 2007; Siegert and Taylor, 2004). I would challenge the question as to whether this really takes place when a client has severe receptive and expressive aphasia, hence the case study at the end of this chapter.

Wressle et al. (1999) found that stroke patients do not often participate in setting goals, which leads to a mismatch of goals between the therapist and client. This in turn leads to the client being dissatisfied with their therapy. Stroke patients' need for respect and dignity is related strongly to their satisfaction with rehabilitation (Mangset et al. 2008).

In many healthcare settings, clients are assessed, SMART goals (specific, measurable, achievable, realistic and timely) are set as required by the medical model in which our services operate and when the goals are met the client can be justifiably discharged. SMART goals (Wade 2009) that are considered to be 'good', because they are specific, might include: 'Kevin will find his way to the bus stop independently by June 1st' or

98

DOI: 10.4324/9781003178613-6

'Sally will identify three types of memory strategy by July 1st'. Such goals are usually identified by the multidisciplinary team in therapy areas of physio, SLT and OT. Smart language goals might include, 'John will be able to order the meal he wants from a menu at his local café by June 2021'. Less specific goals might be 'John will create and use a communication passport'.

There is a great deal of literature about the process of goal setting, why it matters, and how to go about setting joint goals (Davis et al. 1992, Haas 1993, Kagan et al., 2008, Levack et al. 2006, Royal College of Physicians 2012, Sherratt et al. 2011, Ylvisaker et al. 2008, Wade 2009, Worrall et al. 2011). I am not going to discuss the reasons behind goal setting in detail here. The goal of this chapter will be to discuss questions that I have in relation to goal setting with PWA in particular, and whether goals in the general sense of the word should be the focus for therapy with PWA. Based on my own clinical experience, and in line with my preference for taking a more systemic approach to aphasia therapy, I will outline the challenges I see arising from the usual goal setting process and explain my preference for intrinsic goals arising from collaborative therapy.

In neurorehabilitation, where the MDT are involved with the client, attending to physical, cognitive, and psychological changes, goals can be set by the client, with the support of the therapists. Goal setting is often highly dependent on complex language to establish priorities, explain what is possible, negotiate goals, and discuss challenges. With aphasia, however, how are we to explain, identify and work towards goals that are meaningful to the client and their family when that person's language is absent or impaired? In my experience, when language is significantly impaired the goal-setting process is frequently side-lined, and when it is moderately impaired the client plays a passive role throughout the process. In a busy, understaffed working environment it feels too big a challenge, too nebulous, too time consuming, and the client does not make the demands on the MDT that other clients are capable of making. As discussed earlier, PWA often don't have access to MDT input, particularly on an outpatient basis and usually not the neuropsychological aspect, in any setting, due to the presence of aphasia.

I have observed PWA have their goals decided for them by members of the MDT. I would argue that rehabilitation goals are more quantifiable and straightforward to set in the arenas of physiotherapy and parts of occupational therapy, than within SLT when working with aphasia.

Those with severe aphasia in a rehabilitation setting may be informed at the end of 12 weeks that they have achieved their goals, without having understood what those goals were in the first place!

When you have aphasia, being informed of something is not the same as having understood it. This is not to say that identifying goals on behalf of the client is always wrong; indeed, some clients' goals are unattainable or unsafe. Hopefully we listen carefully to the client, regardless of what we think of their goals. However, we are talking about aphasia here, not severe cognitive impairment; by using adaptive communication strategies and skilled listening, there is no reason for the PWA not to participate in the process to some degree.

Who is it for?

Is goal setting more about what is good for the organisation, its administrative systems and/or the funders, or is it about what is good for the client?

The Royal College of Physicians National Clinical Guideline for Stroke (2012) states standards for rehabilitation: 'Rehabilitation must be integrated and context sensitive. Integration will require the delivery of a goal focussed, time-lined rehabilitation strategy.'

I find this statement a little empty and contradictory; can rehabilitation really be 'time-lined' as well as being context sensitive? We also need to ask whether it is the goals that are really driving progress in rehabilitation. As Cooper (2018) states, consciously held goals may be different from those that are actually driving our behaviour.

Work settings demand very specific goal setting as a way of providing evidence of progress to the funding CCG, and for supporting discharge. The course of rehabilitation is often driven by those goals set in the first few days of meeting the client. I have to confess to having been in a situation where I have completed forms with random goals, knowing that these will change once I have got to know the client better. I found the exercise to be rather time-consuming and meaningless; perhaps I am not alone in this experience. The goal-setting exercise early on does not provide the PWA with their basic needs of competence, autonomy and relatedness (Ryan and Deci 2000) that will be discussed below. It doesn't afford them the opportunity to realise what aphasia means to them, to reflect on the impact of aphasia on the contexts of their lives and to come up with more meaningful goals that may be related to wider issues than just language. If a client comes up with a goal which is vastly beyond the scope of their current function (e.g., I want to get back to work as the economic editor) this tells us a great deal about where they are in their understanding of what has happened and about their awareness of aphasia. Setting a SMART goal with this person, such as 'by April I will be able to understand 3-part sentences', may be achievable with therapy, but it may also feel belittling, dismissive of hopes and aspirations, or it will be completely ignored. It is hard to imagine a therapeutic relationship developing from this starting point. Language goals such as this one can be made to fit into the SMART model quite neatly; whether it is meaningful or not is another question.

Haley et al. (2018) offer the FOUR C model for goal setting in aphasia within the life participation approach. Four areas for goals are identified separately: Skills and abilities, Intentional Strategies, Environmental Supports and Motivation and Confidence. This at least encourages thinking about the wider picture when thinking about goals for therapy.

Deborah Hersh et al. (2012) challenged the limitations of the SMART model with aphasia. They proposed a SMARTER framework for goal setting (Shared, Monitored, Accessible, Relevant, Transparent, Evolving and Relationship-Centred). This version of a goal-setting model goes some way to redressing the therapeutic relationship in aphasia to ensure more equality and authenticity; however I do not believe it goes far enough. If the training of SLTs who are going to work with aphasia is still so variable, delivered by educators who have limited long term experience of aphasia (despite having read all the literature), we cannot hope to meet the PWA where they are. The first five chapters of this book outline what I consider to be the core requirements for working with aphasia; it is about the way we interact and position ourselves and what we know about ourselves, that forms the basis for reaching for goals with our clients. With this groundwork the SMARTER goal-setting approach could be more consistently replicated, if goal setting is indeed to be the way forward in the therapy.

It may be true that setting short-term, achievable goals can generate a feeling of success (Locke and Latham 2002), however this does not mean that non-measurable, non-specific goals are any less valuable. Proposing very specific goals may feel reductive and prescriptive to the client who already feels powerless. The family may feel their loved one is not being appreciated for who they are, and their previous competence is not being recognised.

They may even agree to whatever is suggested, rather than question or challenge the ideas we offer which don't seem to fit.

Short-term goal setting does not take into consideration the long-term pattern of recovery from aphasia. If a client is given short-term SMART goals, these are for the purposes of the service provider, and do nothing to let the PWA know that this is only the beginning of a longer phase of recovery, and that there is a lot of hope about the future.

I learned a salutary lesson about recovery even though I had been qualified for 15 years, when I was asked to see Henry. Henry had severe aphasia as well as little insight, cognitive communication difficulties, slow processing, difficulty initiating and finding words, and seemed to wander away from the topic or task in hand at any point. Feeling unable to help Henry directly, I attempted to work with his young live-in nurse/carer on supported conversation. This carer claimed to have had experience of 'teaching' a brain-injured former patient of his to talk again and was convinced he could do the same with Henry.

Due to Henry's marked lack of awareness and the lack of progress with his carer, I discharged him from our caseload. Five years later, Henry's carer had left, frustrated at having discovered that his treatment might not work with Henry after all. A new carer had taken time to understand Henry's background, his preferences and made no demands on him and she approached me again. I was amazed to find that Henry was now sitting in a chair, reading novels, talking in sentences and producing a beautifully intricate drawing every day. We resumed therapy and Henry started to set and complete his own goals, for example staging an art exhibition of his work, visiting specific places in the UK he wanted to see, choosing films to watch at the cinema, designing his Christmas cards. After a further two years of collaborative, context bound therapy he was writing emails, managing some finances and arranging social meetings with friends. In retrospect, I would have taken a different approach with this client, not have been so quick to discharge him, or at least would have suggested six-monthly reviews, had my organisation permitted this.

The achievement of intrinsic (rather than extrinsic goals) is what leads to positive wellbeing (Sheldon and Kasser 1998). This has real implications for how we approach goal setting with the PWA. For example, acknowledging the enormous change and the fear about having aphasia by using supported conversation techniques with the PWA will achieve validation for the client about their experience. Intrinsic to this is 'You are an individual who is suffering. I know you know what is happening and I am listening to you.' This surely is going to enable the client to work towards recovery in a more authentic manner than focussing on an extrinsic goal such as 'You will point to the chart to show what you want for lunch.' (The client who feels safe and heard is likely to work out how to indicate what they want for lunch, when their appetite returns.)

Deci and Ryan (2000) identified three innate psychological needs of the individual: competence, autonomy and relatedness. Exploring clients' expectations of therapy is essential prior to setting goals, as is an exploration of the client's local contexts, relationships and stories. Sometimes people don't know what they want; it takes time, especially after a life-changing event. The same applies to the family of the PWA.

In the case of David, below, his wife observed him achieve a score of 70% on the Arizona test with me (an apparently simple test of linking semantically related pictures). This result indicated significant progress, as a few months earlier I had abandoned the task after three attempts to elicit a response from David.

Far from being pleased, and despite our having established a relationship, she was, of course, distraught. In her eyes, at this point, I was reducing her husband to someone who was only capable of this 'simple' task. I had explained language processing and semantics in as clear a way as I could, but nevertheless she was still grieving the husband who was still here and trying to come to terms with what had happened so drastically to her family. My job here wasn't to cheer her up or give her false hope, however much that would temporarily make me feel better! Instead, I acknowledged her intense sadness at this point, and sat with her while she tried to work out her next steps. Later, I talked to her about language assessments being just a tool to help guide my work, and altogether different from what David 'knows', who he is, who he loves and so on. In other words, I expressed my belief that David was still very much here and asked her to trust me, despite acknowlededging that I didn't have any magic up my sleeve.

Three years on, David's wife understands that his currently ability to understand conversations, make jokes and read news articles was dependent on that development in his recovery taking place. They have worked through enormous adversity, and I have been filled throughout with respect and admiration for them both. As I have been fortunate enough to work with David for this length of time, I have been able to support her and the family through this ongoing process of adjustment, sadness and, increasingly, joy.

103

Had he received 12 weeks post-acute rehabilitation in a residential unit, he would have been discharged at the point when he couldn't associate two pictures together or point to what he wanted, only look blank and passive. Outpatient rehabilitation centres may offer a six eight-week programmes of therapy and ask the client to identify their goals. With aphasia, often the client and their family only want one thing, 'to talk again'. It takes a great deal of adjustment to understand the meaning of the aphasia. By shifting their goals to specifics such as choosing something from a menu, I believe we are taking away hope. Such a limited, linear view only contributes to dissatisfied clinicians, clients and families. Even if we inform families and clients that the goals are changeable, and the goals seem client-centred and rapport established between the PWA, the therapist and the family, there remain many potential pitfalls. These achievements are only seen through our own perspective; the power is still held by the clinician.

Once the goal is written on paper, it becomes fixed; it is somehow harder to alter it, redefine it, broaden it. We as aphasia therapists need to be prepared to shift goals as things progress and change and maybe even question the use of the term goal setting in the context of aphasia.

Intrinsic goal setting in aphasia

In my view, reaching for intrinsic goals with the PWA includes some, or all of (but is not exclusive to) the following features:

Language therapy

A psycholinguistic approach to aphasia therapy is not a process that merely identifies errors and works on those errors until progress is made, as I have heard it described. It may not be helpful to use with some clients. The approach identifies underlying language processing difficulties and then offers a supportive, therapeutic environment where language tasks can be carefully constructed, practised in context and even relatively error-free. This meets the goals of the PWA, which usually include, after all, working on their language. During the course of working collaboratively on language, PWA become more aware of what is happening and why strategies can be helpful. In my view, this work of insight is also part of the process of acceptance and adjustment and gives the client a sense of ownership of their therapy. The intrinsic gains of this work include reduced anxiety, being heard, both of which improve the chances for slowed, deliberate language processing and a greater chance of success. With the availability of excellent tools such as Cuespeak and Step by Step, to devise evidence-based therapy sessions, including home practice to increase intensity, it is essential that our trainee SLTs have a good grasp of psycholinguistic approaches to language therapies during their training.

Demonstrating supported conversation

A systemic view of therapy holds the view that the client (and family) is doing the best they can given the resources they have. A PWA's idea of change and the future may be different from the professional's. Using supported conversation techniques, such as drawing, key word writing, gestures, maps, calendars and so on are the basis for talking about the world as it is, as it has been and how it will be in the future. This process is part of seeing the world differently through talking about it over time (i.e., social constructionism as in Chapter 1).

We discussed supported conversation techniques in earlier chapters. University College London have an excellent resource, for families and healthcare workers, including SLTs. Better Conversations training is available to all on their website (Beeke et al. 2013). Supported conversation is not just a way to communicate with the PWA. Its techniques provide the PWA a way of asking questions, demonstrating competence, requesting clarification, using humour, referring to past discussions and much more besides.

Demonstrating (as opposed to teaching) supported conversation with the PWA for the family, carers, friends and all members of the MDT is essential. To do this I would include the 3rd party in a three-way conversation with the PWA if at all possible. This way you can develop others' confidence with the techniques and show them how to cope when communication breaks down, what to do with silence, how to use pen and paper, and how to sit with the person who might be struggling. If the PWA can only tolerate a two-way interaction, then I would have them observe me interacting with the client in several different situations.

Where I have done this, I have found that communication between the physiotherapist, or OT, psychologist, or rehabilitation assistant can be transformed, and the client starts to build wider relationships of mutual trust with their MDT.

Information gathering

Ongoing conversations with the client and close others, which allow for changing priorities and redefining goals are all essential to a dynamic therapeutic process. Background information questionnaires are undoubtedly useful, as long as we consider past, present and future views about what we hear. In other words, it is important to know what was of interest to them before the brain injury, as long as we consider that interests might be absent or changed right now and may change again in the future. At a point of transition in our lives we are embarking into unknown territory. It is not always possible to enjoy the same things we used to, or we may have to find a way of coping which is different from previous ways we have been used to in other times of difficulty. The systemic concepts of multiple truths and re-framing stories are important so that we can support the client to find their way through this time. Everything that is said should be said speculatively, or tentatively, so that it is never fixed, never irretrievable. It is important to realise that when we explore ideas about goals and the reality of the experience for the client, the client and/or family will help us to select those ideas that fit.

Eliza was a high-performing academic who used to bury herself in work whenever difficulties arose in her life. The sudden arrival of aphasia was particularly devastating, as she was unable to work; she struggled to read and speak. We explored her expectations of the past and the present and this changed her expectations of the future. She could identify her background of wanting to achieve to demonstrate her competence in a male world, and her experience of having been let down by men in her life over the years. She set unrealistic goals which she wanted me to help her achieve. I voiced my uncertainty about these goals, but we set out for them, nevertheless. Being less certain yourself as the therapist allows the client to be less certain and open to alternatives. Eliza was quick to see, through trying them, that they would need to be gradually modified and we did so at her pace rather than mine. Fortunately, I did not have an eight-session limit imposed on my work and she returned to a new academic role.

Sometimes it can be useful to bring the 'former' client into the conversation about setting goals. One way might be to say to the family 'What would the pre-aphasia Michael say to the Michael today about what to do next?'. Such questions are systemic and encourage informed speculation, as the response can reveal many aspects of the client's personality which may not be currently apparent. In addition, it helps the family to adopt a stance they know their loved one would have related to. As Catherine Kohler Riessman (1993) puts it, 'Narrative analysis gives prominence to human agency and imagination, it is well suited to studies of subjectivity and identity.'

Where there is severe aphasia present, as in the case of David, below, I have used the family therapy approach of object use to understand how family members or indeed friends are positioned in relation to one another. By having objects to represent each person, one might ask the PWA to place them according to, for example, who they are closest to at home, who is the disciplinarian in the family, who is the humorous one and so on. Use drawings and objects to reveal how the PWA sees their social context. Partners and other family members, children and friends can join in such a process, which can be light-hearted, serious or just factual. In my experience with people with severe aphasia, this activity can reveal insights into others' behaviours, conversation partner skills, and the effects on the PWA of various physical and social contexts. Sometimes the family are surprised by what the PWA expresses, sometimes it is the PWA who is surprised by what the family experiences since the aphasia has been present.

The therapist can talk about and illustrate differences, positioning of the PWA in relation to others according to the context. It enables people to think experimentally about context and how it might influence the positioning of the pieces.

Miranda was 43, running a successful small business and married to John, when she suffered a stroke. She had mild-moderate aphasia, chronic fatigue, and her speech was hesitant, and she attended every therapy session with her mother, while her 10-year-old son was at school. When I asked about her husband, she was quick to tell me that he is 'not bright' and doesn't understand these kinds of things. She was set on returning to her business, so she could continue to educate her son privately in order for him to do 'better than his father'. When Richard was finally allowed to attend the session with just Miranda, at my request, I asked him about what the experience of the stroke had been for him. The rest of the session became a conversation between the two in which he revealed his great strength of character, loyalty and love for his wife, and how much he valued seeing more of her, and her spending more time with their son. He had observed how their son was happier, despite nearly losing his mother, and was loving having her there at breakfast and suppertime for once. It was as if, in the context of normal home life, Richard had not been visible but now Miranda could begin to reframe her experience of the stroke and not working, from a picture of loss to one of gaining other things. The intrinsic part of this work was that it took away the time pressure to return to work for Miranda with regards her language recovery; she acknowledged that her word finding improved, and she could now start to see and adapt to the patterns to her language caused by fatigue.

Passport or no passport?

A communication passport for the PWA is a bespoke booklet or set of cards which tell their story. It may also include key pictures or names that the person might want to refer to in conversations. Usually devised with the client and the help of the family, it may include a timeline of the person's date of birth, where they have lived, when they had children; in fact any information which seems to be important as reflecting the identity of that person, and which the PWA is unable to express easily for themselves.

Contrary to common misconception, it is not meant necessarily to be used solely by the client to magically communicate whilst the listener remains passive in the conversation. The passport is most useful as providing a starting point for the listener to ask questions from, acknowledge key events, get to know close family and friends, so that the PWA feels heard and understood, if only to a small extent. It must be a shared resource; it might be that a family member needs to prompt use of it to begin with.

Creation of this passport can be a very useful goal, but we should consider who chooses what to put in and what to leave out. How do you obtain the information, from whom and at what point in therapy do you embark on this? Is the person ready to understand the point of having this passport? Do they find it embarrassing? If so, is it the size? The format? The content? Do they just need to experience being supported to use it in various settings so they can experience the positive regard shown by others when there is shared recognition of interest, or place or events?

Someone who had experienced brain injury wrote in a blog online:

Sometimes you do want to know why or who, other times you need to know how. But most of the time you just want to be heard. Not every problem has an answer, questions are often rhetorical, and advice can be a pain in the neck. When we care enough to see someone else's pain, or hear their need for silent compassion, we step out of our cocoon. When we listen quietly we can help them, and ourselves, heal.

Deadlines for goals

In aphasia therapy, we might work for several weeks at a time with little measurable change taking place. Yet the client remains motivated for therapy. On reviewing the situation with the client retrospectively, however, the change seems to have taken place between blocks of therapy. I remember noticing this years ago and feeling very doubtful that my therapy was of any use at all if they did better without it! However, I did notice a kind of 'bedding in' of language and language strategy use.

The PWA also has to find ways to cope when there is no therapy session and falls back on their own resources. Therefore, it can be some way past the identified, specified time in which to achieve the goal, that the intrinsic goals are actually achieved. Equally, work might be aimed at one goal, but result in increased competence in a different area of language where we had not anticipated change. This does not mean the goal is invalid. It shows that we need to be aware that goal setting can be somewhat artificial.

The type of goal set will influence the outcome, and unfortunately the tendency is for therapists to only identify goals which they can achieve in a set amount of time. Personally, I find setting dates by which to achieve goals an uncomfortable process, and I am curious as to why this should be. If I were to say, for example, 'Max will be able to write cheques out independently by July this year', I would only set out to do this if I was fairly sure it would be achieved. (I can only imagine how dull such therapy would be, for me and for Max!) If, however, my goal was 'improve Max's word-finding ability over the next 12 weeks' (not very SMART), the outcome might well be that Max is not only writing cheques, but also making personal phone calls and sending texts, feeling more confident that he has the internal language within his grasp. Additionally, I am working with something I know to be effective (semantic therapy).

When we express uncertainty about how ideas link together, for example, whether using gesture is going to be a useful way to communicate or not, we are permitting the PWA and their family to also come up with and discard their own ideas. Having the opportunity to explore gesture without feeling embarrassment or shame about 'failing' at gestures, for example, is important if we are to move on jointly with the client to alternative interventions. Barry Mason talks about having 'authoritative doubt', or a way of being open to new ideas at the same time as accessing what we know about – in this context, language processing and aphasia.

Dealing with friends

A common experience for PWA and their families is the falling away of friends and what were seemingly loyal supportive friendships. I believe that addressing this issue head-on throughout therapy is an intrinsic part of reaching for the goals of re-establishing friendships and social support. By dealing with it before it happens it can even be pre-empted.

In systemic family therapy clients are encouraged to view other people in relation to themselves. To perceive themselves and their relationships through the eyes of other people. This can help make new connections: between past, present and future: between symptoms and relationship issues: between assumptions and openly held opinions. It allows clients to connect the present with future visions and actions. I use this with people with aphasia, and I explain that they need to educate others on their disability or else people will avoid them. I encourage them to see that what other people fear is losing face when they have a conversation which doesn't go the way it used to. When friends stay away, the PWA feels sadness but also shame. Shame is a significant experience for people following brain injury (Ashworth 2014) and one that we as aphasia therapists do not necessarily consider.

As we saw in Chapter 4, the way we feel about ourselves is closely connected to our behaviour. In my view, friendships are often built on a certain way of interacting, where people play particular 'roles', e.g., John is the one who makes witty jokes, Sarah is the quiet one, etc. and they can become established in a particular pattern of interaction. When someone has a brain injury, friends often feel uncertain about what this means for their social roles with that person. As humans, we are self-conscious and do not like to lose face with others. We also like to solve problems for our friends. When we can't, it is easier to pretend it hasn't happened or to avoid the situation. With our friend who now has aphasia, how can we know what that word means? How do we offer consolation to our friend, what do we do if they can't answer us? Are we going to look stupid and have to walk away without helping? Will my friend be embarrassed when they can't talk back? And how will I get away – I'm so busy, I could be stuck there for ages . . . so I'll just keep away.

The PWA and their family are the ones who need to address these concerns before they become a problem. A goal for the family or client could be to initiate contact with friends. Pre-empt their friends' concerns by telling them it would be nice to just see their faces and know they are there, they don't have to say much, and a very short visit of 15 minutes would be lovely. As time goes on, the PWA may need to share pointers with their friends such as:

I know what I want to say it just won't come out!
Quiet, slow conversations are good.
Please, only one person talk at a time.
Please don't mind a silence, it gives my brain time to think and remember
the word.s
Just seeing you is great.
We can just go for a little walk.

This approach can ensure that absence of friends due to initial embarrassment and uncertainty doesn't become increasingly hard for them to retrieve later on. It also ensures the autonomy of the family living with aphasia.

Self-compassion

The use of compassion focussed psychological therapy (Gilbert 2010) in rehabilitation for acquired brain injury has been successfully used by several clinical psychologists to address the sense of shame and self-criticism that people can experience following a brain injury (Ashworth et al. 2011). Curran et al. (2000) found that self-blame as a coping strategy after traumatic brain injury (TBI) is associated with higher levels of anxiety and depression. Research that looked into men's emotional experiences following TBI found that they can experience significant shame within the social context of their injury. 'Defensive strategies in response to this include self-criticism, avoidance, and submissive behaviour' (Ashworth 2014). We can imagine how this might translate into interactions with friends, so that friends don't know how to sensitively breach these defence mechanisms.

Fiona Ashworth is an advocate of compassion focussed therapy in brain injury rehabilitation. She adopts an 'it's not your fault philosophy' to help reduce shame and self-criticism that people experience post-brain injury

(Ashworth 2014). She describes three types of modus operandi for all of us, one of which might be operating at any one time in our day-to-day existence: 1) a threat focussed state, 2) a self-soothing state and 3) an activating, resource focussed state. People who are more prone to shame and self-criticism are likely to be in the 'threat' state – feeling anger, anxiety, disgust and fear – and may need support to access a resource focussed or self-soothing state and move away from shame (Ashworth 2014).

These psychological difficulties experienced in traumatic brain injury are applicable to many people who have aphasia from any cause, and we have much to learn from psychology about compassionate mind therapy. When the PWA experiences shame, they are likely to push friends away at a time when they most need friendship. Additionally, my observation is that when PWA are in negative emotional states, this significantly interferes with their ability to harness the cognitive processes required in language processing.

I have commented earlier about the historical predominance of men on my aphasia caseload. It has been shown that TBI male service users found compassionate mind therapy exceptionally useful as an introduction to making sense of emotions and their regulation and helping to validate their experience (Ashworth 2014). In my view, it also helps the partner or carer to begin to understand the sense of failure around their loved one's failed attempts to communicate. Ultimately, such an approach might encourage empathy on the part of the PWA for the friends and family who are wanting to support them. Carers too can be supported to learn self-compassion whilst faced with carrying such an overwhelming burden of care.

Can we as SLTs work with psychology to make an aphasia friendly version of such a model? Aspects of compassionate mind therapy ties in well with a systemic approach to aphasia therapy so far described. Early introduction of such a model may influence peoples' capacity to engage in useful speech and language therapy interventions. Together these ideas can preserve and enhance self-compassion, helping those clients with aphasia who struggle to access psychological services to begin to manage the enormous cycle of change that it precipitates.

Recruit support

Cognitive therapy requires intensive training and practice and so does aphasia. Taking a holistic approach to implementing intensive practice involves recruiting support.

Training staff and taking a collaborative approach to this is part of reaching for goals. Staff learn best in the context of the individual that they already know and can relate to, it enables them to reflect on their own behaviour with the client, assumptions they have made, and to explore new ideas around what is happening for the client in interactions, what their thoughts and feelings might be, and what the staff member is experiencing.

With aphasia, it is not easy. You can't attribute the language breakdown to 'cognition' and because the person very likely has intact cognition for the most part, and is often acutely aware of their 'stuckness', it leaves the staff member/carer feeling helpless, embarrassed and sad. Acknowledging these feelings in others is so important. As speech and language therapists we are used to communication breakdown to some extent. Not all carers are, and those who are might have adopted approaches that are either unhelpful to the client, to themselves, or to both. People with aphasia start to be avoided and left alone because it is too hard to converse with them in the ways we are used to. I have seen this time and again.

When working with support staff, I deliberately choose to share my insecurities about whether I am understanding a client or doing the right thing. I want them to know that their insecurities are normal. Family members often feel the same way; it is all part of working with aphasia. When communication breaks down we can still be with the PWA, and be honest about our confusion and our failure to understand. In this way we stay with our trainees, we validate their experience, and they are far more likely to engage with supporting the communication and building a genuine rapport with the PWA. I will have support staff sit in on my sessions and show them how to manage confusion, distress, and how to inject humour when it seems to fit the situation.

I like to make a big issue of how important these poorly paid, poorly trained staff are, to our clients, to us as therapists, and to the families they often talk to. Their role is vital to rehabilitation and clinicians and managers rely on them. Many speech and language therapists will have had the experience of working with an 'amazing' assistant who seems to have natural communication skills. In my view almost every worker can be helped to connect, even in the smallest of ways, when they are encouraged to just be themselves and show kindness.

Maddie was a support worker to Shaun, who had severe global aphasia, with little insight into this. He was in a 12-week residential rehabilitation programme and Maddie was charged with supporting him in the bathroom, dressing and mealtimes, as well as attending group sessions. I noticed that she avoided any interaction where there was not a physical 'task' to be performed.

She was young and shy but clearly very caring. We had a joint session with Shaun where I used his personal biographical book to support our conversation as well as carrying out some Cuespeak language tasks. I asked Shaun about his working life, family and friends, places travelled, interest in cars. When he pointed to 'Publican' and the photos of the pubs he used to run, Maddie's face lit up and she started to tell him she grew up in a pub, like his sons, and as she spoke, I drew diagrams to help Shaun to follow her story. We barely had time for the Cuespeak tasks that I had selected and saved on his iPad, but we completed just one before leaving for the next session.

Following that session, I came across Maddie talking and laughing with Shaun. She had brought in some photos of her pub to show him and he was captivated. Furthermore, she had initiated practising the Cuespeak exercise but also had a go with some of the other exercises on the autorun that I had prepared, and she asked me to check she was doing them correctly.

I would argue that the 'training' of staff is only part of the story; making connections and creating a safe, non-threatening environment for staff and clients with aphasia is crucial to our work.

Dispel the plateau myth

If we use terms like 'spontaneous recovery' or 'plateau in recovery', then our thinking and that of our clients will be limited by such terms. Spontaneous recovery, as I understand it, refers to the impaired aspects of language improving without therapy. In my experience this can happen early on, or it can begin after several months, or barely at all. Full language recovery (even if it occurred) would not leave a person totally unscathed. It would still mean major shifts for the client in how they view the world, their health and their interactions, due to having experienced aphasia.

The word 'plateau' is sometimes given as a reason for ending therapy, and as seen in the example of Richard, above, cannot be stated with certainty. I challenge this notion of 'plateau' from a systemic perspective and firmly believe that individuals have highly variable patterns of recovery, influenced by many and varied factors, which cannot be predicted early on in the rehabilitation process.

Predicting Language Outcome and Recovery After Stroke (PLORAS) is an ongoing study by the Wellcome Trust which is hoping to offer information as to likely prognosis for people with aphasia as a result of particular sites of damage to the brain, by looking at those who are some years post-stroke (Price et al. 2010).

I work with people who have had aphasia for many years in some cases and who are still making progress, long after statutory services have discharged them as having 'reached a plateau of recovery'. Whether or not plateaus and spontaneous recovery are real, positive connotation in rehabilitation is essential. The words we use change the meaning of the problem for those involved. The word 'plateau' does not convey hope. Systemic thinking believes that people have strengths and resources to manage problems and that small changes lead to big changes in life.

Research has found hope, identity and social connectedness to be closely entwined and 'can enable people to both dwell in the present and move towards desired futures'. This research suggests clinicians should prioritise a hope-fostering environment which supports people to develop hope for their future (Bright et al. 2019).

Resistance in therapy

Standard goal-setting approaches, as with many therapeutic interventions, sometimes meet with resistance in therapy. I have heard the terms 'non-compliance' or 'not engaging' used as reasons for discharge when this occurs. Sometimes it is because the therapist has not explained (for example, that using gestures is not necessarily meant to be a permanent substitute for speech, just one of many useful adjuncts to talking). Sometimes it is because the therapist's goals and the client's concerns are out of synch and they reach an impasse. Solution-Focused Brief Therapy offers some useful remedies for this (De Shazer 1985):

1 Complimenting the client and/or family on what they are already doing that is useful and helpful to the person with the communication disorder is essential. There are always small ways that people are doing something well, and I always try to draw their attention to these.

2 Sometimes taking the approach where we 'expand the ordinary' – tell the family what they are doing that is so helpful. I always stress, for example, that they are the only ones who know the client in a unique way, have a shared story with them and no one else can offer their loved one what they offer.

3 Magnifying for family the significance of their role is the backdrop that I feel we should add to our 'better conversations' training for family members. They need to feel useful, and not by being therapists but by being

daughter, son, husband etc. Grandchildren are often reported as being the most skilled communicators by the person in the family with aphasia. 'They don't care' one client told me of his granddaughters, 'they just get on with it and talk to you, tell you what they want to tell you and they observe you very closely, with all the patience in the world.'

Anderson and Goolishian (1988) explain that resistance in (family) therapy disappears when gentler, less power-based therapies are used. They ask, 'Does this mean that resistance is an artefact of the way therapists present themselves rather than as a trait of the family?'. I believe there is truth in this within speech and language therapy with aphasia. Active listening makes room for new things to be expressed and may alter someone's course of action in the face of difficulty. We need to let go of our intentions to influence a client and their family in a particular way, and not equate our own experience with that of others. As Martin Luther King entreats us, we must 'take the person where they are' and put our energies and effort into listening and asking helpful questions.

Allow clients/families to redefine suggestions you make or decide simply that you are wrong. By doing this we start to head towards more authentic goals and the client can be more autonomous. If the therapist still feels strongly that a course of action won't work, they can still offer to pursue it openly and 'experimentally' with the client, supporting the client to make their own discoveries.

Some clients and families, as well as therapists, tend to adopt either/or thinking, which can become a point of resistance. For example, they might be offered a choice of therapy at one session a week or one session a month. We don't live in a binary world; so why have binary choices that are incompatible with our lives? We live in complex, systemic contexts, so consider offering a block of therapy sessions 'to see how we get on'; place the ball for decision about continuation of therapy in the hands of the client, and keep the dialogue going throughout.

'We get as much information when the client does not perform the task as when they do – non-performance is a message about the client's way of doing things rather than a sign of resistance – cooperation with them rather than assigning tasks' (De Shazer 1985). This can also be a feature of successful SLT, when we cooperate with their way of doing things, however small. I would agree with De Shazer when he says that the bigger the goal or the desired change the more likely therapist and client will fail. Brief therapy is different from other therapies, in that no matter how awful and complex a situation is, a small change in one person's behaviour can make profound and far-reaching differences in the behaviour of all persons involved. Only a small change is needed and therefore only a small and reasonable goal is necessary, and this makes it easier to develop cooperative relationship between therapist and client. Personally, I find that when the client shifts from expecting a magic wand, and creatively finds ways to work through things with support, they often make decisions about discharge or intervention goals or sometimes even decide they don't need therapy at all.

I have often been struck by people I have met who, in my view, have severe symptoms of aphasia but don't perceive themselves as in need of therapy. Anecdotally, these are more often older women in my own experience. We cannot assume anything, however. Such people often rely wholly on their own family contexts for support to find a way through and focus on shared meanings and goals.

Case: David

David was 50 and at the height of his career as a prominent journalist, when he suffered a major stroke. After spending three months in hospital, he returned home with global aphasia, affecting all receptive and expressive modalities (i.e., spoken and written language). David experienced cognitive impairments, hemianopia and a right-sided arm and limb weakness requiring him to use a wheelchair. His father and grandfather had died from a stroke at around the age of 60. He had four teenage sons, and his wife Lisa at home.

David has an international reputation within his profession. Prior to his stroke, David's work took him away from home frequently; his lifestyle was not conducive to living healthily for a number of reasons. He had been feeling unhappy about being away from home so much and he used to love coming home and being with his family whenever possible.

David was the decision-maker in the family; a 'larger than life', charismatic person who enjoyed outdoor pursuits and socialising. He had many friends and a wide network of acquaintances. Lisa described herself as a home maker and full-time mother with extended family whom she also cared for. She liked to adopt 'an optimistic attitude wherever possible' and was devoted to her children. Lisa told me that David always valued relationships with people he came across from all walks of life and was particular about politeness and good manners and he always thought the best of others.

I met David three months following his stroke, just after he returned home. Lisa was distraught and exhausted, and trying hard to obtain as much help for him as possible. There had been no psychology input so far, partly due to his severe aphasia, and partly due to the unavailability of such a service in the community.

My initial step was to create a systemic formulation around this family to help me to think about David in the context of his pre- and post-stroke life. The summary below depicts the various aspects of his presentation when I first saw him to consider 1:1 SLT intervention. This framework was helpful to me in that it enabled me to put down all I knew about David and obtain an overview. However, its usefulness was limited to this stage alone, because it would be revised over a period of time.

Intellectual ability

Situational understanding good within limitations of slow processing. Recognises home environment and family, some friends but not all

Executive difficulties

Severe limb and articulatory dyspraxia affecting all output modalities therefore difficult to assess planning/organisation/problem-solving

Awareness

Intellectual – emergent awareness slow
Barriers – family communication style
Adjustment – only to home environment as yet

Attention

Visual and verbal - fleeting or short

Memory

Not assessed

Processing speed

Slow processing speed, impulsivity

Current function

Personal care: help with transfers 1:1 support
Toileting 1:1 support
Cooking n/a
Community access – none
Occupation of time – none
Medication and health 1:1 support

Coping

Resources – family presence comforting
Strengths –willingness to engage, trying to use humour
Challenges –reduced insight

External influences

Overwhelming advice from family and friends regarding his needs

Physical

Fatigue – tolerating 20-minute interactions only
Using wheelchair passively
Right visual field neglect

Mood

Flat, not frustrated, or distressed but some irritability at communication breakdown. Self-discrepancy unclear.

Communication

Receptive: no recognition of written words other than name and limited understanding of single spoken words.

Expressive: limited or no verbalisation, jargon [tu:tu] only.
Social: happy to interact, good eye contact, smiling, not distressed

Current risks

Low mood, falls, children and wife coping emotionally and psychologically

Initially, David presented with relief to be home at last, albeit with flat affect, markedly slow processing, severe receptive aphasia. He relied wholly on others to point and gesture to understand them, with no apparent awareness of comprehension difficulties or his expressive aphasia. David's output consisted of neologisms [tututu] and looking a bit confused as to why he wasn't being understood. He couldn't demonstrate how to use a pen; when placed in his hand he left his hand still and showed no awareness of what to do with it. Pointing and gesture were both absent. He wasn't able to understand a simple semantic task of associating pictures at this stage; or possibly he just couldn't cognitively initiate and execute his pointing responses.

Working directly with David and with the family, I spent time explaining what I understand aphasia to be, using visuals and diagrams. I shared my experience of how recovery from aphasia with different clients amounts to different stories and stressed that David's story would also be unique. I emphasised that the family were already providing David with what he needed most and what no one but they could provide: their presence, their familiarity, a normal home routine and their affection.

It felt right to offer supported conversation training from the start; David was minimally engaged in therapy – he was not responding to simple games (e.g., noughts and crosses) but gradually beginning to show recognition between sessions. This was not at all successful initially. My suggestions were largely ignored, and I felt frustrated by this. The family continued to 'put on a brave face', ploughing ahead with a smile, with their normal style of communicating with one another. Today, three years on, Lisa is a very skilled aphasia communicator. She has developed this gradually over time, and I believe only when she was ready to do so. My role had been to continue to demonstrate the techniques, create a strong therapeutic relationship with David, until it felt safe for the family to make those changes for themselves.

I chose to use the following model adapted from MacDonald (2017) to help me to look at David's communication in more detail and also to track progress where spoken output was extremely limited.

> The model is intended to demonstrate the full range of communication functions and the complex interplay of factors that form an individual's constellation of strengths and weaknesses . . . . The model is proposed as a means of promoting a shared understanding of communication impairment and defining the ultimate goal of communication competence in real-world functioning. The intervention of cognitive-communication disorders is particularly complex and requires analysis of multiple domains of functioning and multiple influences on performance, in multiple communication contexts.
>
> (MacDonald 2017)

This was a useful device for communicating my seemingly vague aims to David and his family. As with many families, their focus was on David talking again and it was hard to explain to them the many invisible cognitive and language processing gains he was starting to make during therapy. My SLT intervention with David can be seen by comparing the two models below of David's communication presentation at the start, and then after a period of therapy.

It is essential that the intention, from the outset, is that such models are revisited and revised at different stages to reflect subtle shifts in progress. The models were helpful in conversations with David and his family about the various aspects of communication to be considered in therapy and at home, and a way for them and myself to identify and reflect on the significant changes despite David still not being able to speak.

From my perspective, the observations made by the family as to David's communication at home were better understood in the context of his cognitive, emotional, physical and communication functioning. Such conversations helped to direct therapy, as well as giving hope for the future as David and his family continued to adapt to the communication disability.

David was happy to be home, enjoying the times when the children were at home providing distraction and laughter, but feeling 'lost' when alone, while his wife was very busy with many domestic and childcare duties, numerous financial dilemmas, and dealing with well-meaning work colleagues, family and friends.

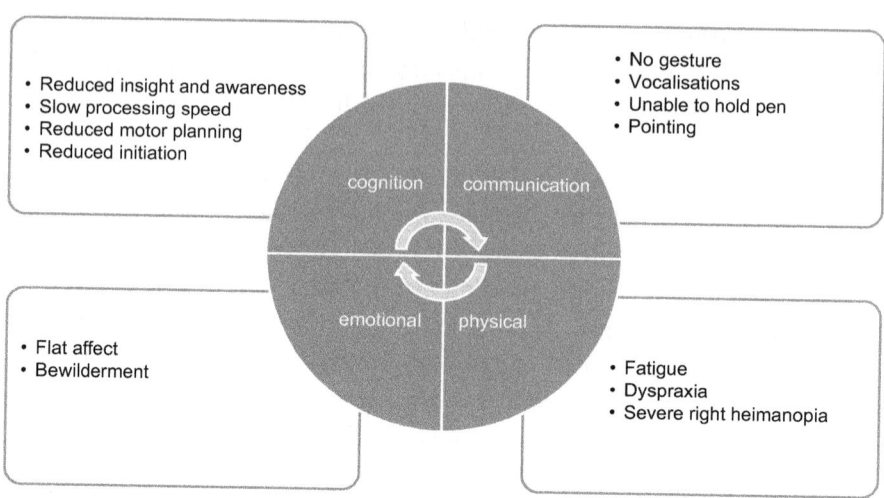

- Reduced insight and awareness
- Slow processing speed
- Reduced motor planning
- Reduced initiation

- No gesture
- Vocalisations
- Unable to hold pen
- Pointing

cognition | communication

emotional | physical

- Flat affect
- Bewilderment

- Fatigue
- Dyspraxia
- Severe right heimanopia

Figure 6.1 Model showing David's cognitive-communication function

Source : MacDonald (2017)

As his cognitive processing ability improved, David showed interest in using his iPad and we embarked together on simple picture, language and cognitive exercises from Cuespeak, Talkpath and Tactus therapy apps. Cuespeak was particularly useful, as it helped him to initiate responses in its question–answer format, giving immediate feedback which helped with the dyspraxia element of his communication. He quickly learned to navigate the exercises independently, and his language comprehension steadily progressed (as did his ability to alter the settings so that he could ensure a 100% score in every task). His interaction with the app was very informative for me in terms of revealing the changing picture of his cognition. There were times when David felt our work was 'too simple', but the presence of topical pictures and current news events in the Cuespeak app helped to make him feel its relevance and have more faith in the process. I reminded David that I was not there to stretch his mind intellectually, only to work on his language processing.

Technological therapies can be worked on with families and carers; however the ideal is for the work to be done with an SLT. The collaborative support of an appropriately trained SLT whilst doing therapy tasks helps to accompany the person and their family through the peaks and troughs which are a normal part of readjustment when one's life has been turned upside down. Sometimes a session might be spent just listening, while the client tells you they wish they had died, that their family would be better off

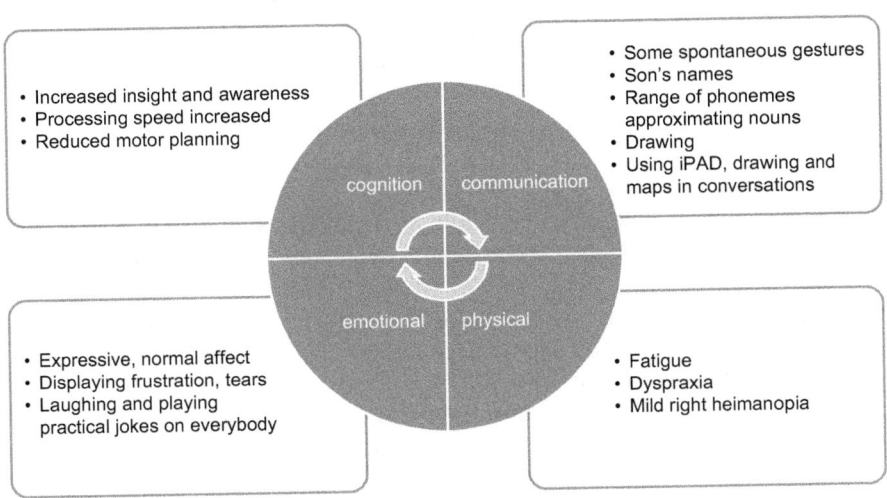

Figure 6.2 Model showing an update of David's cognitive-communication function
Source: MacDonald (2017)

without them; our role is to actively listen and validate the feelings of someone who can no longer express them verbally. Resuming the iPad therapy can then be part of that process.

Figure 6.2 illustrates how the model used at the start can be repopulated to reflect subtle changes throughout the period of intervention, and progress or otherwise in all areas of rehabilitation and adjustment.

Three years on, David was walking, reading, accessing the community, and participating fully in decision-making within the family. Challenges remained, as he was still not able to speak, but his support system had grown around him, and he was becoming a skilled non-verbal communicator.

References

Anderson, H. and Goolishian, H. (1988). Human systems as linguistic systems: Preliminary and evolving ideas about the implications for clinical theory. *Family Process*, 27: 371–393.

Ashworth, F. (2014) Soothing the injured brain with a compassionate mind: Building the case for compassion focused therapy following acquired brain injury. *Neuro-Disability & Psychotherapy*, 2 (1/2): 41–79.

Ashworth, F., Gracey, F. and Gilbert, P. (2011). Compassion focused therapy after traumatic brain injury: Theoretical foundations and a case illustration. *Brain Impairment*, 12(2): 128–139.

Beeke, S., Sirman, N., Beckley, F., Maxim, J., Edwards, S., Swinburn, K. and Best, W. (2013) Better Conversations with Aphasia: An E-learning Resource. Available at: https://extend.ucl.ac.uk/

Bright, F. et al. (2019) Recalibrating hope: A longitudinal study of the experiences of people with aphasia after stroke. *Scandinavian Journal of Caring Sciences*, 34: 42–435.

Cooper, M. (2018) 'The psychology of goals: A practice-friendly review'. In M. Cooper and D. Law (Eds), *Working with Goals in Psychotherapy and Counselling* (pp. 35–72). Oxford University Press.

Curran, C. A., Ponsford, J. L. and Crowe, S. (2000) Coping Strategies and emotional outcome following brain injury; a comparison with orthopaedic patients. *The Journal of Head trauma rehabilitation*, 15(6): 1256–1274.

Davis, A. M., Davis, S., Moss, N. et al. (1992) First steps towards an interdisciplinary approach to rehabilitation. *Clin Rehabil*, 1992; 6: 237–244.

Deci, E.L. and Ryan, R.M., 2000. The 'what' and 'why' of goal pursuits: Human needs and the self-determination of behavior. *Psychological Inquiry*, 11(4): 227–268.

De Shazer, S. (1985). *Keys to Solutions in Brief Therapy*. W. W. Norton.

Freeman, A., Adams, M. and Ashworth, F. (2015) An exploration of the experience of self in the social world for men following traumatic brain injury, *Neuropsychological Rehabilitation*, 25(2): 189–215.

Gilbert, P. (2010) *Compassion Focussed Therapy*. Routledge.

Haas, J., 1993. Ethical considerations of goal setting for patient care in rehabilitation medicine. *American Journal of Physical Medicine & Rehabilitation*, 72(4): 228–232.

Haley, K. L., Cunningham, K. T., Barry, J. and de Riesthal, M. (2018) Collaborative goals for communicative life participation in aphasia: The FOURC Model. *American Journal of Speech and Language* Pathology, 28(1): 1–13. doi:10.1044/2018_AJSLP-18-0163

Hersh, D., Sherratt, S., Howe, T., Worrall, L., Davidson, B. and Ferguson, A. (2012) An analysis of the 'goal' in aphasia rehabilitation. *Aphasiology*, 26(8): 971–984.

Kagan, A., Simmons-Mackie, N., Rowland, A., Huijbregts, M., Shumway, E., McEwen, S., Threats, T. and Sharp, S. (2008) Counting what counts: A framework for capturing real-life outcomes of aphasia intervention. *Aphasiology*, 22(3): 258–280.

Levack, W., Dean S., Siegert, R., and McPherson, K. (2006) Purposes and mechanisms of goal planning in rehabilitation: The need for a critical distinction. *Disability and Rehabilitation*, 28(12): 741–749.

Locke, E. A. and Latham, G. P. (2002) Building a practically useful theory of goal setting and task motivation: A 35-year odyssey. *American Psychologist*, 57(9): 705.

MacDonald, S. (2017) Introducing the model of cognitive-communication competence: A model to guide evidence-based communication interventions after brain injury. *Brain Injury* 31(13–14):1760–1780.

Mangset, M., Dahl, T. E., Førde, R. and Wyller, T. B. (2008). 'We're just sick people, nothing else': . . . factors contributing to elderly stroke patients' satisfaction with rehabilitation. *Clinical Rehabilitation*, 22(9): 825–835.

McPherson, K. M. and Siegert, R. J. (2007). Person-centred rehabilitation: Rhetoric or reality? *Disability & Rehabilitation*, 29(20): 1551–1554.

Price, C. J., Seghier, M. L. and Leff, A. P., 2010. Predicting language outcome and recovery after stroke: The PLORAS system. *Nature Reviews Neurology*, 6(4): 202–210.

Riessman, C. K. (1993) *Narrative Analysis*. Qualitative Research Methods Series 30. A Sage University Paper. Sage

Royal College of Physicians (2012) *National Clinical Guideline for Stroke*, 4th edition. Royal College of Physicians. www.rcplondon.ac.uk/resources/stroke-guidelines

Ryan, R.M. and Deci, E.L. (2000.) Intrinsic and extrinsic motivations: Classic definitions and new directions. *Contemporary Educational Psychology*, 25(1): 54–67.

Sheldon, K. M. and Kasser, T. (1998) Pursuing personal goals: Skills enable progress, but not all progress is beneficial. *Personality and Social Psychology Bulletin*, 24(12): 1319–1331.

Sherratt S., Worrall L., Pearson C., Howe T., Hersh D. and Davidson B. (2011), 'Well it has to be language related': Speech-language pathologists' goals for people with aphasia and their families. *International Journal of Speech-Language Pathology*, 13(4): 317–328.

Siegert, R. and Taylor, W. (2004). Theoretical aspects of goal setting and motivation in rehabilitation. *Disability & Rehabilitation*, 26(1): 1–8.

Wade, D. T. (1999) Goal planning in stroke rehabilitation: Evidence. *Topics in Stroke Rehabilitation*, 6(2): 37–42.

Wade, D. T. (2009) Goal setting in rehabilitation: an overview of what, why and how. *Clinical Rehabilitation*, 23: 291–295.

Wilson, B., Gracey, F., Evans, J. and Bateman, A. (2009) *Neuropsychological Rehabilitation*. Cambridge University Press.

Wressle, E., Oberg, B. and Henriksson, C. (1999) The rehabilitation process for the geriatric stroke patient–an exploratory study of goal setting and interventions. *Disabil. Rehabil.*, 21: 80–87.

Worrall, L., Sherratt, S., Rogers, P., Howe, T., Hersh, D., Ferguson, A. and Davidson, B. (2011) What people with aphasia want: Their goals according to the ICF. *Aphasiology*, 25(3): 309–322.

Ylvisaker, M., McPherson, K., Kayes, N. and Pellet, E. (2008) Metaphoric identity mapping: Facilitating goal setting and engagement in rehabilitation after traumatic brain injury. *Neuropsychological Rehabilitation*, 18(5/6): 713–741.

7 | Endings

Aphasia is usually a long-term condition, despite excellent recovery for some clients. The end of aphasia therapy interventions can be challenging to negotiate for the clinician, the client and the family. Service delivery constraints often limit the number of sessions available and clients and families report feeling 'abandoned', with a sense of shame around asking for more help.

Within my NHS roles, as well as in private practice, I have found that a less linear approach to treatment leads to different, and more satisfactory outcomes. There must surely be a way to translate this experience into NHS provision in order to provide more effective aphasia therapy.

In this chapter I hope to show that a community caseload can operate within a systemic approach, encompassing some of the ideas discussed in previous chapters, as well as thinking differently about discharge in acquired brain injury. The unexpected result of this approach for me, was that I had little or no waiting list, and no longer worried about discharging clients from the caseload. Instead of, as many clinicians fear, an influx of requests for appointments, I found the approach cultivated a sense of control for the client over their own ongoing recovery, in the knowledge that they could have access to support should they need it, as outlined by the National Stroke Strategy 2007.

What's the problem with discharge?

The problems associated with discharge relate directly to the way we embark on aphasia therapy from the outset. This has already partly been covered in this book up to this point. I have found that students and newly

126

DOI: 10.4324/9781003178613-7

qualified therapists, as well as those more experienced (but not necessarily within aphasia) specifically struggle with this stage in therapy. Brumfitt et al. (2005) refer to this in their paper on the curriculum for SLT students. Deborah Hersh describes the dilemma facing SLT's in her paper entitled 'I can't sleep at night with discharging this lady: the personal impact of ending therapy on speech-language pathologists' (Hersh 2010). It has been mooted that students require explicit training in how to manage the discharge process before they even start working.

In 2016, as part of a smaller representation of a focus group of experienced SLTs within the field of acquired brain injury, I presented a talk based on an article entitled 'Factors affecting decision making when accepting clients for intervention and/or discharging from speech and language therapy intervention' (Gravell, Hayden and Palmer, unpublished). This work was based on the need for clarity around the discharge process for students and newly qualified SLTs, concern about making clinical and subjective judgements in an evidence-based world and raising awareness of the multi-factorial nature of decision-making process.

After carrying out a literature search and based on qualitative methods (Glaser & Strauss 1967, Mays and Pope 2000, Charmaz 2006), we identified a range of factors relating to the client, the carer, the environment, the therapist and the service, all of which inevitably impact in different ways on the process of ending therapy. These will not be entered into here; suffice to say that I firmly agree with Hersh (2009) when she says that 'experiences of discharge are best understood in the context of people's biographies, notions of recovery, and understanding of therapy'.

I have outlined below some of the more 'systemic' reasons for problematic discharge that I have encountered, and which I believe would be better addressed from the outset, or in some cases as far back as in student training.

Expectations

Clients and families expect a 'prescription' when they see the speech and language therapists, in line with the medical model of health service in which we operate. The therapist in turn feels 'safe' behind a raft of objective assessments and reports; they don't have to reveal themselves and can maintain 'professional distance'. When it is time for discharge, some clients do not feel heard yet, and as they are not cured, they can feel abandoned.

The SLT can feel despondent when discharging a client, wondering whether their input has been of benefit. The collaborative power-sharing approach to therapy described in previous chapters can reduce, and often eliminate, distress felt on discharge. Looking back over my own career, I can relate to John Steinbeck who once said, 'I wonder how many people I've looked at all my life and never seen.'

If we are talking to clients right from the outset about the process of therapy, and they have the opportunity to be listened to, I find that they themselves know when therapy is drawing to a close. Indeed, my aim from the outset is usually for the client to discharge themselves. I believe this can and does happen if the therapeutic relationship has been good, as long as they know they can come back in the future. When the SLT feels they are nearing the end of therapy, they could ask the client or family if they can start to imagine a time when they no longer need their input and how they will know when that time is approaching.

Dallos and Draper's suggestions about exploring the end of therapy in the context of family therapy might well be applied to the aphasia therapy scenario and could be adapted for that purpose:

- Create a context for a conversation about therapy: Looking back, what has happened for you as a family since we began meeting? How have our meetings been as you expected and/or different?
- Enable clients to review the experience of being in therapy: What has happened to the concerns/worries that brought you to therapy? Are there any ways in which you are different together as a family since we began working together?
- Enable clients to give feedback to the therapist and one another: For my own learning, what would you like me to know about what went well and what I could have done differently in our sessions?
- Clarify with clients that they feel they know how to monitor their relationship and access help when necessary: Are you able to talk with one another about how things are between you and say if anyone feels uncomfortable?

(Dallos and Draper 2010)

Fredman and Dalal (1998) suggest that having an 'open' or 'revolving' door policy reduces dependence on therapy, and that endings can be thought of as 'transitions' rather than a finality. I started to operate an open-door policy and I found that, knowing it was still available was an important resource for clients and that if they knew it was there, they were, on the whole, less likely to use it.

There have been clients where I have tried to show greater belief in their competence by suggesting that they seek further help if they need to 'a few months from now' rather than 'anytime'. If we know our clients well, we will know whether or not the awareness of back-up will support them even if they don't use it. I usually put the onus on them to make the appointment in future. This means that aphasia therapy goes on being a support to our clients, long after our regular appointments have stopped.

The language of discharge

The word 'discharge' means to release in medical terms (OED) but it also means to dismiss, get rid of, set aside or annul. We often feel pushed to discharge clients so that we can offer appointments to those on our waiting lists. Within acquired brain injury, but not specific to aphasia, Leanne Togher addresses the dilemma of discharge, suggesting that discharge is a factor of the model of service delivery and its goal setting approach, as I have attempted to show here. She also emphasises a requirement to facilitate social engagement as part of intervention (Togher 2010), which will be addressed shortly.

Using the word 'discharge' with the PWA or with their family has a finality about it, rubber-stamped by the unwieldy machinations of forms and procedure. If the client waited weeks or even months to be seen, they will worry that re-referral in the future will be just as inefficient.

I was surprised to find that, when I stopped using the word 'discharge' with my clients and families, the process became instantly more constructive. We would discuss when the next session might usefully be, maybe after a few weeks and then months. Often, I was surprised, either by those who I thought were ready to reduce input or by those whom I thought were quite dependent, reaching that readiness much sooner. My waiting list for PWA disappeared when I offered immediate appointments on referral, and an open-door policy on 'discharge', and my passion for the work was reignited.

Fredman and Dalal (1998) write about exploring people's beliefs about endings, in systemic family therapy. Varying discourses of loss, cure and transition in the client's experience, for example, give different meanings to the therapeutic relationship. If at the start of therapy, we think about and situate the person's communication in terms of past, present and future, we are already holding up the possibility of a time in the future when the PWA is no longer attending SLT sessions. Thinking about this point from a safe distance at that early stage helps to prepare the client for when it takes place.

Treacher (1989) (quoted in Rivett and Street 2009) suggest five different types of follow up when family therapy is ending. I believe all of these to be useful with the aphasia caseload:

1   The safety net – a follow-up that provides reassurance in the future.
2   The routine check – a suggestion to e.g., meet again in three months just to check how things are.
3   Telephone follow-up – a short call to the client where things seem to have gone well around discussing discharge, that the therapist is available for a follow-up but they are free to cancel if they do not need a further appointment.
4   Failure follow-up – if the client does not attend, the way this follow-up is done is important, in that it should only aim to inform the client that the therapist is still available. Some processes appear to seek to impose penalty or express criticism about missing the session. If the client does not have a good reason for missing a session (they normally do), I would suggest the problem lies with the therapeutic relationship and needs to be addressed.
5   Research follow-up (I would include the infamous feedback forms etc here): Treacher suggests that this should be planned well in advance of termination in order for it to be beneficial to the client and therapist.

The rescue mindset

We don't often tell clients with severe aphasia that their speech will not recover to its previous level of efficiency, or if we do, we don't support them repeatedly as they gradually begin to grasp this meaning at their own pace.

We operate out of a well-meaning desire to help and relieve suffering; we want to remove all difficulty for the client, but in attempting to do so we can create more challenges and not help them to cope. Perhaps we should reflect on the meaning of human life, which is created through the tensions between, say, sorrow and joy, suffering and achievement and that grief and suffering are a necessary part of experiencing happiness. Truly being with the PWA in this process is the most important job we need to do, in my view.

Martina was a teacher whose severe aphasia resolved steadily over a two-year period. She was highly motivated for therapy and progressed well, determined to prove me wrong and get back to work. Until she achieved this, she said, she would not consider whether to retire or not, even though she acknowledged that her working life had contributed to her ill health. Together we talked about transitions in life, alongside the intense quantity of language work she demanded of me.

I would often receive private calls from her husband who thought she was 'getting worse' at intervals and questioned her cognitive functioning at times. On no account was she to know about these calls, he said, as 'she would be furious' and he declined offers of joint sessions, saying that she would not agree to his being there. I was aware of feeling slightly critical of his behaviour, wondering why they didn't seem to communicate well with one another.

Eventually, the calls ended after a brief exchange as follows: he said, 'I think she is ignoring it, and I don't think she accepts what has happened to her.' My response was intuitive and one of surprise, as I had noticed a huge shift in her mood, acceptance and adaptation to the aphasia, as well as also making good tangible linguistic progress. 'Oh!' he said, 'well, that's food for thought, perhaps it is me that hasn't accepted it, not her.' Martina had not accounted for her family's need to come to terms with her experience as well as hers. She tried to protect them by keeping them out of her struggles. We ended therapy by discussing ways she could help her family to reach the place she had now reached in this process.

Managing uncertainty

We are not good at dealing with uncertainty in our own lives, so we don't know how to talk to the PWA and their family about uncertainty around the level of language recovery and the time that it might take. Much distress at discharge is around this ongoing uncertainty for the client and managing this potentially without the support of the SLT (after all there is no psychological support available either).

Learning to manage uncertainty for the clinician, the client, as well as the client's family can be liberating when we consider different types of certainty.

Barry Mason (1993) offers a useful framework for thinking about this, and one which allows more flexible thinking around living with uncertainty:

'Safety' = emotional, physical and psychological containment.
'Certainty' = knowing about the condition to be treated and the means of doing so to lead the client to a better place.

From these two concepts, four different combinations can present themselves, according to Mason (1993) and as described by Dallos and Draper (2010):

Safe certainty – the therapist knows what to do to help me.
Safe uncertainty – the therapist will try to help but is not quite sure how and I will have to be active in this.
Unsafe certainty – when people do not feel contained but there is a pressure to be certain, for example to generate a diagnosis or grasp at a solution.
Unsafe uncertainty – the sense of being overwhelmed by the complexity and enormity of the problems and not knowing where to go and what to do.

Our clients often look for 'safety' in the context of the 'certainty' of health services, but this does not really exist in real life; we can never be totally certain and totally safe. Safe certainty about the future, even if possible, would inhibit growth and even lead to poorer mental health in the long run. The SLT who gives the client the belief that they offer safe certainty, will run into many problems when the end of therapy approaches. If we feel unsafe and certain we are unsafe, we are likely to feel very helpless, angry, upset, and look to blame external things for our predicament.

A place of unsafe uncertainty is indeed a fearful place to be, and sometimes dealt with by trying to control the smallest things within our environment, e.g., by behaviours, to bring about a scrap of certainty. Our role as aphasia therapists is to embrace the uncertainty and empower our clients and their families to move from the overwhelming 'unsafe uncertainty' and the helpless 'unsafe uncertainty' to a position of 'safe uncertainty'. In order to do this, Mason advocates adopting 'authoritative doubt' with the client, or offering therapy solutions tentatively, in order to share the position equally, as I have discussed previously. As he says, 'We own expertise in the context of safe uncertainty. Relational risk taking involves owning your own position and taking risks in order to get some safe uncertainty' (Mason 2005).

The way therapy goals and tasks are presented will affect the way our clients deal with uncertainty about future outcomes. If we talk about recovery or solutions, this suggests there is a final goal to be reached. However, even in brief solution-focused therapy, de Shazer and Berg (1988) hold a constructivist stance which sees dilemmas as ongoing, rather like a river – aphasia can be viewed like this too.

We must not forget that our work, especially where there is severe aphasia, is also about the position of the carers or family members and friends, 'Families often entertain safe and unsafe uncertainty about whether they are good enough carers or are doing the right thing in the professional's opinion' (Baum et al. 2011). In systemic terms, it can be helpful to use therapeutic curiosity to find out more about how the family makes sense of its situation (Cade 1995). In the context of aphasia therapy, this relational risk-taking enables us to take a metaposition of imparting knowledge but at the same time creating an environment where knowing and uncertainty hold equal weight for us and for the client/family. I am aware that my practice shifted in this way some years ago. In positioning the client and the family as the experts as to what fits them best, from what I have to offer, I noticed greater 'engagement' in sessions by clients, as well as by their families, who often just want to know if they are doing everything that they can do to support their loved one.

But I'm not a counsellor

We are often constrained in SLT by the linear view that 'counselling' and 'speech and language therapy' have boundaries that we must respect; I have yet to hear a clear description of what these boundaries might be and I am certainly not convinced by them. I do acknowledge, however, that currently SLTs are not adequately equipped to deal with the complexity of aphasia. If counselling is distinct from SLT, what happens to the PWA when, as is currently the case, counselling is only available to those without aphasia?

As a speech and language therapist I particularly like the quotation by Hayward (2003), 'If we accept that language creates our perspectives as well as reflects them, then different language practices will be required to access different perspectives and to think outside of what is routinely taught'. We can apply this both to clients who have experienced change, loss and communication impairment as well as to the actual language practices that are possible with people with a language impairment, i.e., finding alternative ways to communicate, using visual resources to back up speech, using diagrams, gestures, props etc. I agree with the view that accessing expert knowledge (e.g., about language disorder), can emphasise that dysfunction is a property of an individual rather than a problem to be re-storied (Lock et al. 2005). In the context of narrative therapy White et al. (1990), say that people organise their lives around specific meanings and thereby inadvertently contribute to the survival of the problem. I think this is true. In the case discussed below, Gerry's dominant narrative was that his articulation needed to be accurate for him to know he had improved; through the process of aphasia therapy this dominant narrative slowly changed to one of connections, relationships, meanings and self-confidence. When this begins to happen, many difficulties can be addressed, through the SLT process, and not necessarily through separate counselling.

What happens next? I still need therapy!

Sometimes clients will say that therapy has not helped them. Nevertheless, they spontaneously take on responsibility in navigating the minefield of communication with their families in their own way, and can be determined to find work etc. Sometimes a PWA may not have insight into their aphasia, or they will know they are not communicating with others but cannot hear and alter the jargonistic words they are using. In such circumstances it is all the more important to offer support to the family system, and not end the sessions because you can't cure the aphasia.

Geoffrey experienced such aphasia but with no physical disability. He would talk to anyone during his stay in the rehabilitation centre, at great length and with expressive intonation and emphasis, using only jargon (nonsensical words). He would sometimes come to the office and sit and recount things that had happened to him in his life – stories filled with humour, shock, love, pain; the emotions of which I had no trouble gleaning, but I couldn't tell you what the 'plot' was. For many weeks he was preoccupied with thoughts of his wife deserting him, of dying and being buried, he pointed to the ground repeatedly and his wife described a long history of depression prior to the stroke, in which he often had suicidal thoughts. I wondered how on earth I was going to manage the discharge conversation with his wife the week he was due to return home. There was no local SLT service available to him and he had made no progress with speech. On the day of departure, Gina came in dressed to the nines, with a suit for him to wear. She thanked me (I thought I had done very little) and said that Geoffrey had turned into the loving, attentive husband that he used to be many years ago. She said that she had agreed with him that she was going to retire early; they were just going to go home, rebuild their garden with a large pond and enjoy spending time together again. She did not even mention the availability of community SLT services. Gina and Geoffrey's story was unique to them and they were choosing to do what fitted with them at this stage in their lives. To me, in my context of work, Geoffrey had many and severe impairments; to his wife he had regained the characteristics she loved and which had been lost for many years.

Together with one of my clients, I set up an aphasia café in my local town in order to further support clients with aphasia, as well as their closest family. Located in a publicly accessible café, its aim is to encourage PWA to go out independently, perhaps on the same day as visiting the bank or post office, with the purpose of meeting and interacting with people. This model is in practice elsewhere in the UK, but groups vary in the ways in which they operate; some are more 'directed' by an SLT, some are run by PWA only as support groups.

Our cafe became both an integral part to delivering the 'ending' of aphasia therapy within the community and giving clients the opportunity to decide for themselves whether individual sessions were still required (see Gerry below). The owners and staff at the café were told about aphasia and began to experience for themselves an element of what PWA are living with. They began to breach the barriers that PWA often feel are there when trying to express themselves in public.

In such an environment, aphasia is diminished, while relationships, laughter and stories of accomplishment come to the fore and are enhanced. This reinforces the aforementioned meaning of community 'to support one another to be the best they can be' when they are ready to step outside of the cocoon of their home or therapy clinic.

Having started up two of these cafés, and according to many of those PWA who attend, I think the presence of an experienced SLT is essential. Many SLTs do not understand the reasons for this and set up cafés to run independently as a support group. This is perfectly valid, but my point is that such a group plays an altogether different role in the process of ending therapy from the model I have used. Indeed, I have found that a regular outcome of the café has been that members meet up independently anyway as they form natural friendships. It is not only a stroke group either; PWA following stroke, brain cancer or any other aetiology for the aphasia are invited to the cafe following a period of therapy or on discharge when they are ready to move on to getting on with life with a communication impairment. In café sessions I have experienced a member who caused distress by expressing racist views, another who tried to insist that 'victims' sit on one table and 'carers' sit on the other. As an SLT, experienced in thinking about communication challenges, and seeing things through the eyes of PWA, I was able to avert distress, and maintain an open, supportive environment for everyone. It will not always be possible for the person with aphasia to do this and still be supported by the group; I accept that others may disagree with me.

The expertise of an SLT in aphasia lies in facilitating discourse, where aphasia of varying severity is present, enabling conversations, responding to concerns of partners if they also attend, ensuring inclusion, and, most importantly, ensuring the competence of the PWA is revealed. These skills are underestimated, and often by our own profession.

The client will order and pay for their own refreshments and join the group at any point within a two-hour period. Freedom of choice in this latter aspect is vital, in a collaborative approach, as I believe there should be no controlled beginning and end to the group, people should be free to drop in and out at will. It is all part of maintaining an equal relationship. The SLT sits with PWA and their close others, clearly demonstrating, incidentally during conversation, new ways of 'talking' (e.g., using pen and paper, drawing, slowing speech etc.) so that understanding can be created between people and for individuals as they interact.

Gergen (1985), Shotter and Gergen (1989) talk about the 'interpretive and hermeneutic approach to understanding therapy'. Meanings are co-created during conversation; people are not just 'information processing machines' (as extreme adherence to the cognitive model might suggest). Through spending time at the café PWA and their partners explore experiences of transition and adjustment, they become a panel of experts for one another, and encourage reflection on their own progress, and what the future might hold.

As mentioned repeatedly, the National Stroke Strategy, and the life participation approach call for practising participation and providing long term support for PWA. Using a café this way provides educational, psychosocial and economic benefits but it is rarely available as part of a community service. I found that the presence of the aphasia café meant that people always had access to an SLT for questions, or factual expertise, and they frequently decided after attending the café that 1:1 therapy was no longer needed.

Observations from café meetings after many years now are that news is shared, good and bad but always with a good dose of humour. Members visit and meet one another on other occasions, often helping each other out. Laughter is the predominant feature of the group. New members are included immediately and welcomed by regular members.

Validation of one another's struggles, achievements and personalities is invaluable in the adjustment of PWA to living with aphasia. Members greatly value one another's comments and feedback; they expect positive regard by the SLT, but positive regard by group members is optional, making it that much more valued. Everyone can be included, regardless of severity of aphasia, as total communication strategies, and repair or coping strategies are regularly demonstrated by the experienced therapist with individuals concerned and this gives others the confidence to interact with that person.

For the PWA the café provides the following:

- the opportunity to express hopes and frustrations
- support for others, including relatives, as well as receiving it – affirmation, confidence, humour
- demonstrated use of supported conversation in natural conversational setting
- reduced anxiety and depression
- a natural communicative setting
- countering loneliness and isolation
- allowing limitless possibilities if so wished
- sharing experience of happier times
- finding humour in current difficulties
- revealing aphasia to public setting by involving café staff and educating on aphasia
- empowerment when 'expert' members with aphasia can support new members
- sharing between different age groups of participants, which may include children during holidays
- discussion about recent developments in software/therapies, research.
- Shared experiences.
- Enquire about other people's lives – empathising with and supporting others

This model of ending therapy clearly has benefits for the service, the client and the clinician.

As we have seen, a systemic view of change is one called safe uncertainty and is not a fixed position. New explanations can be placed alongside those that the client and therapist bring and help people to see that solutions don't always solve things. Family therapist Cecchin (1987) famously said that 'when the family cures itself of being sick and the team cures itself of the idea of being useful – that is the ending'.

Case: Gerry

Gerry was an editor for a news publication in the city. He was fit and well and starting to reduce his working hours in anticipation of retirement, which was fast approaching, when his speech became slurred during a phone call to his daughter one evening. Thanks to the media publicity on TV to act FAST, Sarah knew to call an ambulance and he was in hospital within half an hour.

Gerry recalls that although everything was a blur, he could see his daughter at his side and 'she was talking "gibberish"'. Wanting to ask her what on earth she was talking about, he found he couldn't utter a word. He suddenly felt 'unreal' and disorientated, and a scan confirmed a significant stroke. After a physical assessment by the doctors, Gerry was back at home by the following afternoon. His daughter, who was a self-employed mother and also running a business, offered to stay with him for a few days, as the 'only' impairment observed was his aphasia, which was characterised by severe stuttering when attempting to talk. He was not allowed to drive.

Fortunately, a referral was promptly made the same day to the community service where I worked and by Monday afternoon Gerry was sitting adjacent to me with a cup of coffee, looking every bit as anxious and panic-stricken as I would expect, given the weekend's events. Gerry expressed concern that 'the words don't come' and when they did, they stuttered out incoherently. He was under the impression that the faster one acts, the quicker one will recover from all effects of a stroke. I immediately imagined the variety of advice he might have been given at the hospital by different health professionals; he had not been there long enough to have been seen by an SLT. Gerry's daughter waited outside; in retrospect I would have invited her in, although she was anxious not to trample on her father's need for autonomy, in this as in many other situations in their day to day lives.

Language assessment using relevant parts of the Comprehensive Aphasia Test showed that Gerry had mild-moderate receptive aphasia, mild-moderate dyslexia, and severe expressive aphasia with neologistic errors, semantic errors, word initial hesitations, prolongations, imprecise consonants and disrupted stress patterns on polysyllabic words.

Feeling that Gerry wanted to understand more, I wrote down key words and used arrows and shapes to link ideas together visually. I drew a head with a spiral of spaghetti in the brain region, illustrating how his stroke had caused a blockage that is permanent, and in the region where words are stored. Brain plasticity was explained simply, reassuring him that 'diversions' around the brain can be developed, which is why we see progress over a longer period of time. I explained that each person with a stroke is different, and his journey will not be identical to anyone else's, but that I would support him through the process. I showed him how the rest of his brain was unaffected and therefore I recognised that he could think, remember and 'know' things as usual. Like most PWA, he needed to know that 'I know that you know'. I noticed that Gerry started to relax, and as he did so I noticed he was starting to understand more quickly as well as find his words more easily.

Each time I saw Gerry in those first few weeks I explained the same three things that as SLTs we know intuitively but forget to talk about overtly. It becomes 'obvious' to us, through familiarity, but we must always 'meet the person where they are' and take the time to clearly share what we understand to be true. It is hard to retain unfamiliar information especially when you have aphasia and especially when you are also struggling to function differently in a world which has stayed exactly the same.

Firstly, his stroke had only just occurred; his brain needed time to settle down and begin its physiological recovery. We were in a post-acute phase, which is very early days, and many people who have had a significant stroke will be in hospital for days, weeks or even months. The FAST acronym (face, arms, speech, time) refers to the urgency to obtain medical treatment for a stroke. Prompt action can make the difference between a patient receiving the right treatment or not, but aphasia takes time to resolve. Thankfully, he is where he is now, safely home and with support, and I urged him to allow himself time.

Secondly, his processing speed was slower than usual as his brain is still physiologically trying to recover; I showed him how, when I spoke slowly and gave him time to process, his understanding on the tests I gave him was markedly better. I pointed out that while his thought processes are going at full speed, fuelled by anxiety, his language lagged behind and therefore speech needed to be slowed right down to match that pace. Through repeated demonstration Gerry began to be reassured that this did seem to be the case.

Thirdly, I told Gerry that I have seen others with similar, or worse aphasia, and things never stay the same at this point; possibility for change is ever present and that I would support him through this process. All I considered to be certain was that he would not recover his speech 100% as it was before, but we would work together to get it as near to that as possible. I have found that clients appreciate honesty and directness delivered with kindness, above blind reassurances that they will get better delivered with sympathy. Gerry was a man with an academic background, having studied history before becoming a journalist. I warned him that our work together would involve seemingly simple tasks, viewed through a lens of literary academia, but that I was not here to stimulate him intellectually – I would not presume to be able to do that. My role was merely to help him to access the *language* which he still had in his brain, through structured practice.

Gerry attended SLT sessions twice weekly for six months.

Therapy targeted word retrieval. His reading ability already permitted the use of written words, short sentences as well as drawings. Gerry was given time and structure to process meanings in a given context.

Initially tasks included selecting words belonging to an identified semantic category, adding items to these by drawing, completing sentences with a missing word. The semantic bias of the carrier sentence was gradually reduced, as his success grew, so that he began to deal with increasing competition for words in his internal lexicon. Gradually Gerry began to spontaneously write words down (albeit with many spelling errors which we disregarded initially) the focus being on finding the right word in any form. I stressed that things being right or wrong was not the point in the work we did together; it was the process of doing that mattered; the process of joining up the dots. Gerry enjoyed tinkering in a workshop with his car enthusiast friends, we had practiced names of tools, car parts and repairs that were a new world of words to me.

Gerry's language and speech steadily progressed to reading on his computer, instructions, letters and all functional reading tasks; he could talk to his family on the phone to relay information, ask questions and make plans. He became more relaxed about doing the tasks we had set together and started to 'forget' to do them. He continued to be susceptible to fatigue, his speech was still dysfluent, and the words didn't come easily when he wanted to have a conversation. We looked at how much progress he had made, and I persuaded him that ongoing recovery would take place, at a slower pace most likely.

I suggested to Gerry that therapy was coming to an end. He didn't agree. Gerry continued to contact me for more appointments, and I reiterated what I said at the start, that he couldn't expect to return to his former language function 100%. He arranged to see me and asked me whether he should pay for private therapy on a daily basis to make further progress. Instinctively, this didn't feel like the best solution for him at this stage in his recovery, but I felt stuck and unsure how to help further. Relative to some of my other clients he could do so much and had lots of support. What I didn't consider, and would now consider first and foremost, was his very personal need for autonomy, his struggle to come to terms with the changes, and his fear about the future.

Gerry was the divorced father of four daughters he had largely raised alone. He lived alone but kept a close eye on his children and grandchildren, teaching his grandchildren to bake and learn to manage their finances during holidays while their parents worked; his role was one of head of an ever-growing family; he had raised them through great adversity in his own life and they were doing well. The loss of speech threatened this role far and above not being able to work or having to retire earlier than planned.

It was at this point, feeling rather helpless, that I talked to Gerry about a communication group at the therapy centre. We invited others and sat round a table with coffee. I tried hard to encourage participation; everyone was friendly and seemed willing but remained passive, wanting me to structure the group. It felt inauthentic to me, and most attendees were dependent on being driven or arranging transport to attend; the whole process felt like dependency and that is not what I had envisaged at this stage.

Lanyon et al. (2018) found that PWA evaluate the benefits of group participation against factors such as transport, distance, consistency of location and facilitators the presence/ absence of close others and relationships with services/ speech pathologists.

I decided to adopt the aphasia café idea, using the approach I have described above. The effect I desired for the group occurred instantaneously. When people arrived at the café one by one, or with their partners, ordered their drink and chose a place to sit, conversation immediately flowed. It was my turn to take a passive role, as I could barely get a word in edgeways!

After only a few weeks of attending the café (for the full two hours each time) Gerry said that he realised how far he had come and that the best thing for him to do now was just to use his speech as much as possible. Having an SLT available in the context of the café group was still very important for him, but he no longer wanted 1:1 sessions.

Seeing Gerry's response to the café, I collected the views of other participants over a period of time. Comments by PWA who attended the café included:

'without the café you would still feel very much on your own following the stroke'

'I like seeing people, chatting, with similar experiences, otherwise you'd be on your own'

'even though you've got better, it's nice seeing everyone get better still'

'different conversations help to broaden your vocabulary and the things you talk about'

'it's good to be with people like you, the cafe is quiet, and comfortable'

'people teach me how to speak, I catch up on gossip and there are younger people as well as older ones'

'I I like the friendship element; amongst friends there is no need to apologise for your speech'

'the cafe is a positive thing as everyone is in the same boat'

'we really missed it over Christmas . . . wondered how everyone was getting on.'

Some relatives joined the group, but I always encouraged them to take time for themselves and leave the PWA there if they wanted to. It feels important to show compassion for carers as well as clients, and not criticise their choices. I did not want people to stay out of obligation, and often it was better for the PWA to have the opportunity to speak for themselves. When relatives talked too quickly or without sufficient consideration for the PWA, I gently pointed this out and modeled more helpful ways of talking and interacting. Many relatives benefited from the indirect conversation support training they inadvertently received, and I observed their interactions with PWA change over time. They reported;

'It's nice to see how other people communicate with their partners and I can use those ideas with John'

'I've noticed younger SLT's learn a lot from the talking to people in the cafe'

'You can feel isolated as a carer, so we get the same friendship and support from the group (as our relative with aphasia) – it's a real tonic'

During the recent global Covid 19 pandemic, the aphasia café has been meeting online. Although a better substitute than not meeting at all, it has been evident that, for those who live alone, speech can deteriorate through lack of use. Meeting again in person allows this to improve when lockdown restrictions are lifted once more. Online cafes only allow one speaker at a time, and it is public to the group, whereas in the natural environment, people have the opportunity for several conversations, some private, and a greater range of topics, with different people.

Gerry is now an expert on his own aphasia, and still very much the head of his family and offering advice and help to his wider network of friends. He still struggles with his speech, particularly if he has not spoken for a few days, but several years on he is still available to support new members joining the weekly café and has since earned the nickname 'The Chairman'.

References

Baum, S., Gray, G. and Stevens, S. (2011) *Good Practice Guidance for Clinical Psychologists when Assessing Parents with Learning Disabilities*. The British Psychological Society.

Brumfitt, S. M., Enderby, P. M. and Hoben, K. (2005) The transition to work of newly qualified speech and language therapists: Implications for the curriculum. *Learning in Health and Social Care*, 4(3): 142–155.

Cade, B. (1995) John H. Weakland (1919–1995): Tribute to a pioneer. *Journal of Family Therapy*, 17(4): 357–362.

Cecchin, G. (1987). Hypothesising, circularity and neutrality revisited: An invitation to curiosity. *Family Process*, 26: 405–413.

Charmaz, K. (2006) *Constructing Grounded Theory: A Practical Guide through Qualitative Analysis*. Sage Publications.

Dallos, R. and Draper, R. (2010) *An Introduction to Family Therapy. Systemic Thinking and Practice*. Third edition. McGraw Hill.

De Shazer, S. and Berg, I. K. (1988) Constructing solutions. *The Family Therapy Networker*, 12(5): 42–43.

Fredman, G. and Dalal, C. (1998). Ending discourses: implications for relationships and action in therapy. *Human Systems: The Journal of Systemic Consultation and Management*, 9: 1–13.

Gergen, K. J. (1985) The social constructionist movement in modern psychology. *American Psychologist*, 40: 266–245.

Glaser, B. G. and Strauss, A. L. (1967) *The Discovery of Grounded Theory: Strategies for Qualitative Research* Aldine de Gruyter.

Gravell, R. Hayden, S. and Palmer, H. (2016) Unpublished presentation to the 2016 Royal College of Speech and Language Therapists Annual Conference, 'Factors affecting decision making when accepting clients for intervention and/or discharging from speech and language therapy intervention'.

Hayward, M. (2003), Critiques of narrative therapy: A personal response. *Australian and New Zealand Journal of Family Therapy*, 24: 183–189.

Hersh, D., (2009). Breaking the connection: Why is it so difficult to talk about discharge with our clients with aphasia? International Journal of Speech-Language Pathology, 11(2): 147–154.

Hersh, D. (2010) I can't sleep at night with discharging this lady: The personal impact of ending therapy on speech-language pathologists. *International Journal of Speech-Language Pathology*, 12: 283.

Hersh, D. and Cruice, M. (2010) Beginning to teach the end: the importance of including discharge from aphasia therapy in the curriculum. *International Journal of Language & Communication Disorders*, 45(3): 263–264.

Lanyon, L., Worrall, L., and Rose, M., (2018) What really matters to people with aphasia when it comes to group work? A qualitative investigation of factors impacting participation and integration. *International Journal of Language and Communication Disorders*. doi:10.1111/1460–6984.12366

Lock, A., Epston, D., Maisel, R. and Faria, N.D., 2005. Resisting anorexia/bulimia: Foucauldian perspectives in narrative therapy. *British Journal of Guidance & Counselling*, 33(3): 315–332.

Mason, B. (1993) Towards positions of safe uncertainty. *Human Systems*, 4: 189–200.

Mason, B. (2005). 'Relational risk-taking and the therapeutic relationship'. In C. Flaskas, B. Mason and A. Perlesz (Eds), *The Space Between: Experience, Context and Process in the Therapeutic Relationship* (pp.157–170). Routledge.

Mays, N. and Pope, C. (2000) Assessing quality in qualitative research. *BMJ*, 320:50.

National Stroke Strategy (2007) Department of Health, UK. Available at: https://nsnf.org.uk/assets/documents/dh_081059.pdf

Rivett, M. and Street, E. (2009) *Family Therapy: 100 Key Points & Techniques*. Routledge.

Shotter, J. E. and Gergen, K. J. (1989) *Texts of Identity*. Sage Publications.

Togher, L. (2010) The dilemma of discharge and some possible solution. *International Journal of Speech-Language Pathology*, 12(4): 320–324; discussion 329–332.

Treacher, A. (1989) Termination in family therapy – developing a structural approach. *Journal of Family Therapy*, 11: 135–148.

White, M., Wijaya, M., White, M. K. and Epston, D. (1990). *Narrative Means to Therapeutic Ends*. W. W. Norton.

8 Aspirations for aphasia therapy

This chapter will look at some of the suggestions in current circulation for effective aphasia therapy approaches, and critically analyse them through the lens that a systemic approach would offer. The limitations of these suggestions, with reference to systemic literature, will be discussed as well as their many affordances. The case of Angus and Sandra at the end of this chapter includes lists of 'impairment therapy' tasks that I used with Angus. They are not explained in great detail, as that is not my intention for this book. The reason for including them is to show how language therapy can be interspersed with a more family therapeutic approach in aphasia therapy.

A reconsidered, universally agreed and focussed approach to SLT training in aphasia that considers the specific needs of the PWA, and their families is advocated. In my view it is urgently needed.

I have supervised many students and graduates of SLT courses who are unprepared for the clinical reality of an aphasia caseload. They express doubt in their ability to offer effective interventions for this client group, and feel overwhelmed by the linguistic, cognitive, emotional and psychological complexity of what they encounter in the client and their families, and how it impacts them emotionally and psychologically. Many will be drawn to the objective rigour and structure of postgraduate dysphagia training, and only some years later some will express curiosity again about the adult acquired communication caseload. I would argue that this is because they have by then matured, have some clinical experience elsewhere and therefore feel comfortable expressing their uncertainties. Surely the time has come to address the incongruity of available training courses when it comes to offering sound aphasia therapy training?

DOI: 10.4324/9781003178613-8

In Chapter 4, I explained what drew me to this profession, and the personal experiences which have the potential to make me either a very poor therapist or a very good one. Being able to understand and reflect on this has enabled me to be alert to how I interact with clients and their families and given me the confidence to approach and deconstruct difficult topics.

All SLTs have their reasons for joining the profession, indeed they are normally asked this at interview. We need to understand that these personal narratives have a far-reaching impact on our work. We know that PWA do not access psychological services, and that the SLT is often the person who is hearing enormous psychological distress. Students of aphasia and cognitive communication impairment after brain injury, arguably need to be supported in this *before* they reach the clinic.

Best practice recommendations: Aphasia United

In 2011, the idea of an international organisation to drive change by 'uniting the global aphasia community through a strategic plan and shared vision' was conceived at the Clinical Aphasiology Conference in Fort Lauderdale, Florida. I was interested in this as soon as it came about, having worked with PWA in Tanzania and through Swahili language in the past and being very aware of the global inequity of services for this population.

Aphasia United is made up of experts in aphasia and has developed best practice recommendations for healthcare and community services involving people with aphasia (www.aphasiaunited.org). These recommendations are available in an increasing number of languages and also in aphasia-friendly versions of these and can be seen on the website. I support most of the recommendations wholeheartedly, and acknowledge they are 'best practice'. Sadly, such terms often get interpreted, as 'we would do that if we had the resources, but we don't, so we can't'. I am not sure such a view is valid across the board. Why can't we start off with best practice, albeit with limited resource?

I would suggest that implementation of these recommendations in the UK, given our current aphasia SLT training, is a long way short of the mark.

People with aphasia should be offered intensive and individual-ised aphasia therapy designed to have a meaningful impact on communication and life. This intervention should be designed and delivered under the supervision of a qualified professional.

(Aphasia United)

Unfortunately, there appears to be little consistency of belief in our training institutions about which skills the qualified professional should have, and even less consistency in what they do turn out to have in practice. Evidence-based research used to back up teaching approaches is not exemplified by good quality practice-based evidence. Excellent clinical practice does not necessarily find support in research literature. For example, a student may learn about the efficacy of sematic therapy but find themselves working in a setting that does not support that approach, and therefore discards such ideas from their toolkit.

People with aphasia should receive information regarding aphasia, aetiologies of aphasia (e.g., stroke) and options for treatment. This applies throughout all stages of health care from acute to chronic stages.

(Aphasia United)

The latter part of this statement is of huge importance, and yet it is rarely translated into our models of service delivery in community services in the U.K., which limit themselves to a few sparse sessions following six weeks' highly variable early supported discharge provision. Managers are still telling their SLTs that only a finite number of sessions can be offered to PWA.

What about the quality of those sessions? A few excellent sessions are far better than many poorer quality ones, where the client is coming back again and again with unanswered questions. What about the skill set of the therapist? What constitutes a session? Is there an aphasia café locally? There are so many variables, and while the lack of resources (e.g., insufficient numbers of SLTs in the community setting) needs to be addressed, it does not fully explain the reason for the lack of quality therapy on offer.

Distribution of SLT services is grossly inequitable (an acute hospital in my region employs 30 SLTs in adult services (13 WTE = working time equivalent), while the local community serving that trust employs 2 WTE). It would be useful to have national figures as to how many SLTs work in acute settings compared to community, and how many work with aphasia compared with how many work in other areas of adult services nationally. The Royal

College of Speech and Language Therapists was unable to provide this data at the time of writing.

We cannot expect SLTs to want to work in aphasia therapy if we do not adequately equip them to do so in a way that is appealing, supportive, and enriching and which also aims for professional autonomy. A well-trained aphasia therapist does not need to be told how many sessions to offer, or indeed how to manage their caseload efficiently. Sometimes, the aphasia therapist's job is to 'do nothing' and to just listen; truly active listening is an acquired skill, not just a friendly chat.

My own experience is that my training and clinical experience, with the support of an aphasia-friendly manager, and transformed further by the systemic training, has enabled me to use limited resources effectively. I enjoy a richly rewarding and fascinating profession, and one which could be available to many other SLTs with the right support. PWA and their families would reap rich rewards from a fresh approach to aphasia therapy.

> No one with aphasia should be discharged from services without some means of communicating his or her needs and wishes (e.g., using AAC, supports, trained partners) or a documented plan for how and when this will be achieved.
>
> (Aphasia United)

Whilst I endorse the sentiment behind this recommendation, I believe that in the absence of a systemic approach to aphasia therapy, we can only provide a very reductive service. Without advanced skills in asking questions that truly reveal the PWA in the context of their lives and help them to identify their own route to adjustment, we are in danger of making assumptions about what kinds of 'needs and wishes' those might be, as well as about whether the trained partners actually understand and use their skills in practice. The result of missing the mark in this way is that we end up with long lists, dependent clients, unhappy families, uncertain students and exasperated managers.

Asen et al. (2004) suggest that questions about the wider context which the patient is part of can be seen as interventions in consultations. Questions can be more important than answers, as asking the question can alter ways of thinking about the difficulties for the client and the therapist. For example, carefully asking a PWA about their desire versus their ability to communicate with others can be quite revealing. I learned to ask questions that I thought I already knew the answer to, only to find that actually I was wrong. We all tend to assume, and I for one have often assumed wrongly. Asking questions compassionately, that take into account the guilt and shame people experience, is vital. Asking questions in a way that engenders self-compassion. Curiosity about somebody's reasons for cutting themself off from others may reveal surprising answers. Don't assume you know. Asking in detail about their experience with aphasia; what, why, when, who, how questions are useful. I have seen 'poor historian' written in the medical notes of a hospital patient with severe aphasia, as if the blame for not telling their story should be on the person who has lost their language, not on the lack of skilled questioning by the note-writer.

The reference in the best practice recommendation above to AAC (augmentative and assistive communication) as a first suggestion fills me with anxiety in the context of the PWA. I realise that AAC can refer to many different devices, but none of them can ever be a substitute for the language processing in the brain. For me, as for many aphasia therapists, the days of handing out pictorial communication charts with multiple images as a panacea to PWA are behind us. And yet, people who cannot grasp what aphasia can possibly be, who are recovering and distressed, are *still* given a sheet of images of a toilet, a newspaper, a urine bottle and similar, which they cannot see the purpose of, cannot scan adequately and worst of all, feel silenced by, because it removes the burden of really understanding and of active listening from the staff member.

The use of iPad and similar in aphasia therapy has revolutionised our work; I have discussed the fantastic linguistically creative features of Cuespeak. TalkPath and Tactus apps can also be effective if used selectively, with therapist support and adjusted for individuals. Yet these are not communication aids. Health workers and families seeing us use them think they might be, we need to explain what we are doing.

I have lost count of how many times a relative or a medical worker has implored me to find the right 'gadget' for the PWA. They look at me in disbelief when I say it doesn't exist. Working with aphasia is not the same as working with people whose motor speech is impaired. There is no point in fudging our response to this question – we have to be blatantly honest if we are to encourage people to work at their aphasia. Personally, I have known only one PWA out of the many hundreds I have worked with, for whom a Lightwriter was a helpful adjunct to her communication. Even in her case, however, it was no substitute for pen and paper in conversations, where properly supported conversation could take place. AAC puts the onus back on the PWA and discharges others from their responsibility to become involved. Pens and paper are ideal; they are cheap and never need charging, and that is why they are often overlooked.

> *Intervention might consist of impairment-oriented therapy, compensatory training, conversation therapy, functional/participation-oriented therapy, environmental intervention and/or training in communication supports or augmentative and alternative communication (AAC) . . . Communication partner training should be provided to improve communication of the person with aphasia.*
>
> (Aphasia United)

As indicated above, I think it would be helpful to leave out the AAC and be more explicit about supported conversation practice. I have carried out supported conversation training in many establishments, with many family members, I have shared Connect's excellent series of published resources (Connect.org is no longer operational) and I have referred people to the free Better Conversation training tool provided by UCL. And yet, in spite of having attended training, I hear support staff say, 'but that doesn't work with x' or 'I still think he understands everything I say', or 'he wrote down f.i.g. so I bought him some figs but he threw them on the floor. What else can I do!'

Supported conversation is a dynamic process, and the individuals involved in any one conversation are all different. Nowhere do people learn the purpose and meaning of supported conversation better than with an individual client *that they already know*, and with the modelling of a skilled SLT.

> *Families or caregivers of people with aphasia should be included in the rehabilitation process. Families and caregivers should receive education and support regarding the causes and consequences of aphasia.*
>
> *Aphasia United*

Training videos of clients one doesn't know do not have the same effect, in my opinion. PWA are so different, the trainee does not easily translate one person's presentation to another's, and why should they?

Showing how it works in a real context, with a specific client, and supporting the health worker to do the same, develops the skills and confidence of the health worker far more effectively. With continued discussion with the SLT, they will gradually start to apply their skills to new clients in creative ways and start to form their own problem-solving techniques.

It is as much about using a power-sharing, collaborative systemic approach with our health workers as with our clients. This way they are far less likely to reach for the antiquated communication board.

The Seven Habits of Highly Effective Aphasia Therapists

The Seven Habits of Highly Effective Aphasia Therapists are expressed as a set of values or habits that define effective aphasia therapists, from a 16-year programme of research by Professor Linda Worrall of the University of Queensland. The project sought to capture the perspectives of people with aphasia, their family and speech-language pathologists (Worrall 2019). These are very welcome in my view, as they go a long way to encouraging a person-centred approach to aphasia therapy. Worrall et al.'s 'seven habits' are discussed here, with reference to how a systemic approach might develop and enhance such habits.

'Prioritise relationships'

Worrall et al. define the effective aphasia therapist as having 'relationships as a philosophy of practice'. This is basically true, but I don't think it goes far enough. A true philosophy about relationships requires an understanding of how meaning is created through social interaction, how the self-impacts on such social constructs. This has already been discussed in the earlier chapters of this book.

Alan Carr (1998) lists four key insights which are central to practice within family therapy and which we might consider as part of our relationship philosophy of practice in aphasia.

I   patterns of interaction within the family and the wider social network may predispose family members to have problems or maintain these problems once they occur.

II family life cycle transitions and crises may precipitate the onset of problems for individual family members.

151

III therapy which involves both the individual with the problem and significant members of the family and social network is an effective approach to ameliorating many difficulties.

IV such therapy is not haphazard but is guided by certain hypotheses about the most useful way to proceed.

I believe SLTs are often in a position of offering haphazard therapeutic support because they are not trained in useful techniques for helping families to cope.

Curiosity and neutrality are considered by Cecchin (1987) to be some of the key qualities of effective therapists working with families; if the therapist shows curiosity and flexibility the family is more likely to question its own beliefs and behaviours. The therapist needs to be able to ask questions that don't necessarily reflect their own viewpoint, whilst simultaneously taking into account everyone else's views. Conceptually, the therapist needs the skills to be able to think about relationships in terms of multiple levels of meaning, action and context. This includes seeing themselves as an observer who influences what is being observed.

'Find a rope team'

I agree that aphasia groups are social microcosms and are vitally important in our communities. In the UK, stroke groups are more likely to be available than aphasia groups. Those who do not understand aphasia, might consider stroke groups to be adequate substitutes. They are seen as serving a wider membership and being more cost effective. I disagree, they are not a substitute, and would stress the need for aphasia-specific groups.

We saw in Chapter 7 that aphasia groups vary in their design. I am not sure I agree with Lanyon et al. (2018), who say that the aphasia group needs to have 'structure, and group objectives'. For me, such a framework immediately imposes structure on what should be a natural communication environment. Group objectives, in my view, should be general, for example sharing experiences, supporting one another and so on. A skilled aphasia therapist will be able to facilitate an authentic context in which individual and group objectives can be shared, reached and reformulated as they evolve, experienced as part of group membership.

New members should be permitted to bring new ideas and objectives; these need to be incorporated in a fluid way that responds to the dynamics of the group. A new member will of course influence the group as a whole, and this too is part of the practice for the PWA in meeting and communicating with new people who may have with greater or lesser severity of aphasia symptoms than themselves. Shared roles or responsibilities are needed within 'the rope team' but only to the extent that individuals want to share; this will alter over time, as people adjust to living with aphasia. Negotiation of this requires skills that are too easily overlooked.

'Begin with the end in mind'

As discussed in Chapter 7, the ending is determined by the beginning. Worrall et al. quite rightly emphasise the importance of 'knowing what the end can look like'. However, as previously discussed, SLTs don't have adequate training in this, or in knowing when the end might be approaching, and what it means to 'live successfully with aphasia'. How does the inexperienced therapist support clients in how to navigate the acceptance and otherwise of friends when they have aphasia? Is it about giving advice or is it really more about carefully listening and asking the questions which will enable the person to find their own solutions?

Kyla Hudson refers to two themes in living successfully with aphasia, which are 'doing things', and 'other people'. In my view, a systemic approach aims, not for the PWA to be doing specific things necessarily, such as shopping, or joining a group, or activities. It is more about the PWA getting to a place where they can begin to *feel* like doing things. Most PWA will find a way to do the things they want to do, but sometimes need the therapist's help to find the will, as well as to carry hope for them until they reach the place where they can carry it for themselves.

'Practise SMARTER therapy'

I believe smarter goal setting needs to be firmly based within the therapeutic relationship for it to be meaningful and engaging to the PWA. It also needs to take place at the right time, led by the client and not driven by an external framework imposed on services. The PWA may not be ready to order a taxi, if they are still confused and filled with questions about why they can't talk and whether they have 'lost their marbles'. Worrall et al. (2019) advocate therapy planning *after* goal setting so that therapy can be goal-led. Systemically thinking, and in my practice, there is no prescription about goal setting and therapy planning, as the intervention would be therapist-and-client led.

'Leave no person behind'

It is encouraging to hear the drive to actively support PWA to the next phase. This also means that being actively involved in mental capacity assessments where someone has aphasia. PWA are excluded still in many decision-making scenarios and in all phases of care; acute, rehab, and community. Mental capacity assessment in aphasia is a book-worthy topic on its own; for the purposes of this discussion, however, just a short example follows:

Mark was aged 50. We already had a good therapeutic relationship from therapy sessions in the past, and he contacted me to ask me to accompany him to an appointment with a consultant psychiatrist. His GP had struggled to understand what Mark had been trying to tell him about managing his diabetes. Mark had become frustrated, resulting in the GP referring him for a psychiatric assessment. Living alone by choice, Mark prized his independence and privacy above all else and had no close relatives; I was astounded when he told me the GP thought a psychiatrist was needed.

Fortunately, Mark was able to reach me and asked me to meet him at the psychiatrist's consulting room. He wanted me to tell the psychiatrist that he was fine, he was attending the aphasia café, as well as all his diabetic nurse appointments, and that he didn't want any extra assistance at home at this time but would let his GP know via the SLT if this changed in the future (Mark had recurring meningiomas that required neurosurgery from time to time). The psychiatrist looked totally bemused by Mark's aphasia, and our ability to communicate comfortably using supported conversation. The consultation consisted in Mark reassuring her that he was not suicidal, and that he knew what he was doing. We left the interview in good humour, Mark having irreverently made several funny jokes at the psychiatrist's expense.

I knew that Mark had capacity to make decisions. He sometimes travelled alone across country, navigating complex train changes, and he managed his home and finances, but his communication meant that he was continually being left behind by the services around him, merely because of his aphasia. I contacted the GP to offer my support for any future medical consultations if Mark needed and consented to that support.

'Look behind the mask'

Low mood has consistently been shown to affect quality of life and the ability to live successfully with aphasia (Cruice et al. 2003). The majority of people with aphasia will have depression (Worrall et al. 2016).

A guide for NHS commissioners (NHS Improvement 2011) identified needs for Psychological Support for Stroke. Unfortunately, very little mention was made in that document of the significant proportion of stroke survivors with aphasia and how provision for them might have to differ from that of the general stroke population.

It is estimated that, at the point of discharge, 25% of stroke survivors on an acute stroke unit will have ongoing need for psychological /counselling support. A significant proportion of these psychological difficulties remain undiagnosed or inadequately treated (Hackett et al. 2005). If untreated, according to the aforementioned document, this can reduce the impact of rehabilitative interventions, resulting in impaired physical functioning, a longer duration of rehabilitation, increased long term institutionalisation and long-term care and higher mortality rates. Depression affects about 30% of stroke survivors and can happen any time after the stroke event (Hackett et al. 2005). People with aphasia and impaired language skills (expressive and/or receptive impairments) are likely to suffer continuing difficulties with psychological adjustment beyond six months and therefore require ongoing psychological support. Mood disorders are associated with worse outcomes in the longer term, including increased morbidity and mortality (House et al. 2001; Pohjasvaara et al. 2001).

Stepped psychological care in stroke was proposed as a framework for supporting people after a stroke (NHS Improvement 2011). We must remember, however, that figures obtained in relation to stroke only account for some of those we meet with aphasia. Many people have aphasia as a result of injury, surgery and disease. In this model (Fig.8.1), levels one and two can be provided by non-psychologists, but with the supervision of a clinical psychologist, whereas level three requires specialised intervention.

Caroline Baker (2017) points to effective therapies offered to PWA in Level 1 such as biographic-narrative therapy, communication partner training, aphasia choir, self-management workbook and goal setting. In Level 2, psychological education and problem-solving with therapist support is advocated, possibly using techniques provided by psychological strategies training where it is available.

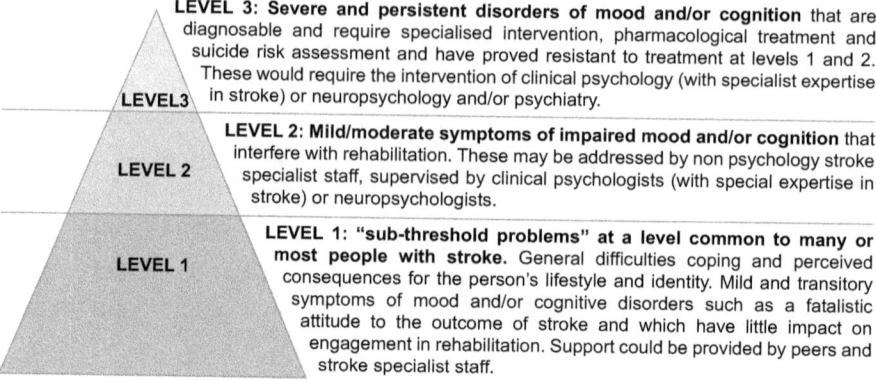

LEVEL 3: Severe and persistent disorders of mood and/or cognition that are diagnosable and require specialised intervention, pharmacological treatment and suicide risk assessment and have proved resistant to treatment at levels 1 and 2. These would require the intervention of clinical psychology (with specialist expertise in stroke) or neuropsychology and/or psychiatry.

LEVEL 2: Mild/moderate symptoms of impaired mood and/or cognition that interfere with rehabilitation. These may be addressed by non psychology stroke specialist staff, supervised by clinical psychologists (with special expertise in stroke) or neuropsychologists.

LEVEL 1: "sub-threshold problems" at a level common to many or most people with stroke. General difficulties coping and perceived consequences for the person's lifestyle and identity. Mild and transitory symptoms of mood and/or cognitive disorders such as a fatalistic attitude to the outcome of stroke and which have little impact on engagement in rehabilitation. Support could be provided by peers and stroke specialist staff.

Figure 8.1 Stepped psychological care in stroke was proposed as a framework for supporting people after a stroke

Source: NHS Improvement (2011)

I have completed the training in Coping Strategies Post-Stroke specifically for the stepped care model, using a combination of CBT and solution focussed therapy approaches, as well as attending train the Trainer sessions, designed to enable us to roll out the training to other health workers. Having attempted this, I would maintain that it is wholly inadequate for our clients with aphasia. Aphasia barely gets a mention in the training, other than to make reference to mood screens purportedly standardised on PWA. It remains a prescriptive, medical model, which is not tailored to the unique concerns of the PWA and family. Further, I have never worked in a community setting where clinical psychology support is routinely available to me for my interventions. A systemic therapeutic approach as described so far in this book would better equip the aphasia therapist to support all levels, 1–3. I would propose that specified circumstances would then be identified that would require joint working between a clinical psychologist and a specialist aphasia therapist to support the individual and their family.

Narrative therapy approaches are just one aspect of a systemic approach that have a lot to offer the aphasia therapist in 'looking behind the mask'. Todd and Weatherhead (2014) have written about narrative approaches in the context of brain injury; 'Narrative therapy techniques and their underpinning philosophy are intended to reduce the impact of any given problem by helping the person to develop a perspective on her experience of life, which is not wholly consumed by the problem. It cannot make the brain injury go away, but it can stop a person feeling wholly defined by it'.

The systemic idea that we can 'Think differently about being different' (Swain and French 2008) connects with the notion that narratives are not just reflections of identities; they *constitute* identities. 'Narrative therapy concerns itself with the deliverance of clients from the weight of oppressive and totalizing stories by liberating the client's voices and preferences' (Doan 1998).

According to Michael White (1998), three sets of factors constitute lives and identities.

1   The meaning people give to their experiences or the stories they tell themselves about themselves.
2   The language practices that people are recruited into along with the type of words these use to story their lives.
3   The situation people occupy in social structures in which they participate, and the power relations entailed by these.

PWA are silenced in respect of these elements of personal narrative by the services which claim to treat them. We know that 'people are unconsciously recruited into the subjugation of their own lives by power practices that involve continual isolation, evaluation, and comparison' (White 1998) and our job is to help them to deconstruct these elements. In addition, we can assist them in deconstructing assumptions and practices that her unhelpful to them. As Worrall et al. (2011) point out:

> Impaired communication acts as a filter between the participant with aphasia and health professionals, blocking or hindering them from obtaining or accessing appropriate information and services. Therefore, during stroke rehabilitation, those patients with aphasia may be additionally disadvantaged and dis-empowered.

PWA are not given the opportunity to negotiate new identities with the support of a person who is skilled with aphasia and also has appropriate psycho-therapeutic training. As I have referred to earlier, my experiences suggest there are male-female differences in the take up of such support. Male clients in particular seem to benefit from external support which is beyond the confines of their families in this respect. Male clients are the ones who mostly attend the aphasia cafes. Extreme self-criticism can be an aspect of depression, as we saw in compassion focussed therapy, as can an overwhelming sense of powerlessness, anxiety and fear about the future. As previously stated, but nevertheless important to reiterate, systemic and/ or narrative therapy is collaborative, but the client is the expert in their lives (Murdoch 2009). This philosophy contributes a great deal to empowerment in supporting the PWA through depression.

Nancy Murdock (2009) describes many useful ideas, some of which we could certainly apply to our work in 'looking behind the mask' in aphasia therapy. As a systemic practitioner, I have received training to use many of these, and frequently do so in my work in aphasia:

- Talking about different 'ways of men being' for example, rather than the one way this person knows and lives.
- Anthropology– a commitment to grounding people's stories in cultural and historical contexts.
- Social constructivist approach. The way we view ourselves and others and the social world we live in is created by social processes and through our interactions with others.
- Social power (Foucault in White and Epston 1990) – the person is political. Clients are encouraged to question the dominant stories of their culture, so that therapy is a kind of social or political action (White and Epston 1990).
- Feminist values of demystifying therapy – commitment to making therapy as transparent as possible and also a stance against oppressive practice and questioning structures where men have a dominance and power in relation to women.
- Awareness of the western concept of individualism, which is not so powerful in other cultures.
- Dominant stories are rich and thick; alternative stories tend to be thin: the therapist's role is to develop or 'thicken' these alternative stories.
- Problem-saturated stories restrict the view of the person and don't include their strengths and competencies – How we behave in a situation is influenced by the most dominant story at that point in time

(Zimmerman and Dickerson 2001)

'Find a voice'

Recognising that people with aphasia and their family are the most effective advocates for better aphasia services is indeed important. As is supporting

PWA to advocate for better services. However, I would also warn anyone with aphasia as well as SLTs that not everybody with aphasia wants the same thing. Neither are they affected by the consequences of the aphasia in the same way, nor do they experience it the same way. We must all remain open to hearing about individual differences.

Clinical research: my challenge

My own career has been characterised by an on-off relationship with clinical aphasia research. I have become somewhat irreverent towards aspects of aphasiology research that seem to divorce language dynamics from human behaviour, but at the same time I feel frustrated with the widespread lack of consideration for psycholinguistic processing in the university and clinical settings. The evidence base for many language-based therapies seems to me to be devoid of the all-important therapeutic relationship and the therapeutic relationship approaches seem to be devoid of any understanding of linguistic processing.

Service pressures for ever more 'efficient' practice in order to save time, data collection to account for every minute spent at work and endless mandatory training for every conceivable eventuality result in clinicians looking for guaranteed treatment solutions and quicker fixes. Aphasia therapy sits uneasily within these models of practice. I have been aware of a reduced desire in recent years among supervisees to read and digest recent studies in the context of clinical practice and my allegiance swings with ever greater momentum from evidence-based practice towards practice-based evidence, the more I uncover complexity in my work and find new ways of working.

Rivett and Street (2009) talk about the skills of the good therapist, in systemic therapy terms, as being in their ability to monitor and maintain the therapeutic alliance in spite of all the obstacles and problems of everyday practice. I would echo this in the context of aphasia therapy, where the challenges of communication, family relationships and past narratives can all present as challenges to negotiate. In clinical linguistic research, these messy aspects are eliminated, and I agree with Roth and Fonagy (1996) who state that 'There is a risk that the sophistication of research trials that demand clear causal influence can overregulate therapy content and underemphasize the freedom of action available to individual therapists.'

The clinical aphasia therapist has the job of applying the wide-ranging findings of research across a variety of areas to their work with individuals. No easy task to replicate without the constraints of the research design. However, 'It is in the application of the general to the individual that marks out the skilful clinician' (Rivett and Street 2009) and we need to equip our trainees to do this adequately.

Case: Angus and Sandra

Sandra telephoned me one day. On answering the phone, I could hear sobbing as she struggled to get the words out, 'It's my husband, and he's had a stroke. I don't think you can do anything because they told me at the hospital just to go home and rest, but it's awful, he's so angry, I don't know what to do.' I invited them to visit me the next day.

Two weeks earlier, Angus had been driving home from his daughter's house at 1 am. He almost stayed the night there after talking at great length to the family about some ongoing wider family concerns but decided to get home for some rest. He had not been drinking, after all. He explained that he was stopped by a police patrol car on the way home for driving erratically. He described trying to tell the officer there was something wrong but being unable to speak coherently. When the breathalyser test was negative, he was taken into custody for further drug testing. Whilst in a cell, he was ordered to tie his shoelaces and he found he could not move his right hand adequately to do so. He tried to tell the officers he needed help but couldn't say anything or work out what to do to get his meaning across. His head was pounding, and he felt trapped in a nightmare. It was only after some time that another officer came in and noticed his face had drooped, leading them to discuss whether to call an ambulance.

On admission to casualty, a CT scan confirmed a stroke, with right-sided body weakness and 'mild aphasia'. Angus was released from police custody and discharged home the same day with a raft of medications and advised to see his GP as soon as possible.

On appearance, Angus looked entirely normal; his right-sided weakness had mostly resolved. He nodded and interjected in his wife's conversation appropriately, 'yes, that's right', 'thanks', 'in here?', 'Oh ok, that's fine'. When I asked him about his family, however, he asked me to repeat many times and in response he strung numerous words together in a sentence-type format which conveyed no propositional content.

Angus and Sandra attended 22 sessions in total. They carried out a great deal of practice in between first weekly, then fortnightly sessions. A simplified outline of the work we did together is represented below. From the start I was very hopeful about Angus's recovery. He and Sandra did not feel hope at that point, far from it, but in holding hope for them we were eventually able to share it properly, as Angus moved forwards.

After the first few sessions, Angus hit a very low point, emotionally and psychologically. Our conversation in that session where I used systemic-style questioning allowed me to understand more about Angus the person, the family man, devoted grandfather to a severely disabled little girl, his fears and his need for a sense of control in his life. From that point onwards, we touched on these things repeatedly, but the dynamic altered; Angus himself took responsibility for his therapy and worked towards discharge. In the end, he seemed to know when the time had come to end our sessions.

Initial sessions

Angus presented with fluent jargon aphasia, empty phrases, with a mixture of English jargon and neologisms arising in part from phonological errors. Some sentences conveyed meaning with some attempts at self-correction, but awareness of jargon was variable. He always asked for repetition and looked carefully at my face and lips to aid his understanding. Sandra was upset and tearful. I have summarised my initial findings here:

- Moderately impaired auditory comprehension in conversation, (increasing to severe when fatigued) aggravated by impaired auditory and phonological processing.
- Easily overwhelmed by rate of speech, complexity, amount and duration.
- Auditory word – pic matching (Palpa) 37/40 – errors all corrected on repetition (auditory processing difficulty)
- Reading aloud – 20 words, some sounded out and ? comprehension.
- Confrontation naming 18/20 but very stressful for Angus.
- MOCA 23/30 (errors only in auditory processing)
- Verb test – auditory comprehension – 27/30 – errors purely auditory processing
- Newcastle verb comprehension part 1: 25/32, however 32/32 when verb written down. Angus showed good comprehension of verb once processed into semantics from phonological input.

161

- Wrote down words said aloud: horses, Tesco, London, names of family.
- Picture description: 3 verbs, 14 nouns, no overall scene setting, paucity of content words naming errors (semantic) and automatic phrases e.g. 'rubbish . . . on the TV' Able to be more specific with prompts, absence of sentence structure, tendency to list,

> *obviously windows.. computer ..going through TV ..whatever it is .. photo..something eat the telephone..rubbish on the TV ..no bin ..eating the burger ..somebody the time ..somebody popping the door... pen ..crayon obviously a drink stuff there...that's it...*

> (The picture used from the MCLA assessment (Elmo et al. 1995) shows a man sitting before a computer at an untidy desk, with a window cleaner behind him, a burger on the desk, wastepaper everywhere and somebody poking their head round the door.)

Fatigue was a big challenge for Angus and yet he was pushing himself hard to do better. He would become very frustrated and angry with Sandra when she didn't understand him and then regret making her cry. I lent Sandra the Connect book entitled *Better Conversations* (no longer in print) and suggested using writing, gestures and drawing to communicate. I advised Angus to stick to 1:1 conversations and not with the wider family at this stage. Short tasks and rest periods were suggested, reassuring both that there were many strengths in Angus's current ability that gave me hope that he would continue to make progress over time. Informing them about the aphasia café I run gave them the idea that there would be support in the longer term. The fact that they never chose to take it up did not matter at all.

Therapy sessions and practice tasks

- Writing nouns under categories (written word association too simple!)
- Phrase generation from a noun – too hard (labelling nouns, with no verb generation)
- Verb pictures – challenge to pare down to core semantic verb rather than list associated nouns. Angus became very anxious with this task – errors and poor self-monitoring increased frustration.

We talked about his progress and increasing difficulty of tasks as part of that. I found that he needed lots of reassurance. He was reminded of leaving school at 14 and associated bad memories regarding academic attainment. I reiterated that I view language and intellect as separate and that we were working to re-access the language his brain has already acquired, not to start from scratch.

- Subject-Verb-Object pictures – helped him to access the verb but noun retrieval so much quicker he often replaced verb with nouns still
- Suggested naming things and actions through the day (Reduced Syntax Therapy (Springer 2003)) and charades with his wife to identify actions.

One day, Sandra told me Angus was not keen to come for the session. I was glad she felt able to let me know this. He had brooded over the challenge of the previous week's session despite my reassurances and his mood had been very low over the weekend. I suggested we meet for a conversation rather than therapy that day. They were both tearful and we talked about the trauma of experiencing a stroke, how he feels his brothers pressure him into talking when he craves peace and quiet.

Angus's realisation of the effects of the stroke was growing and he felt angry and upset. As the session progressed, he became more relaxed. We talked about what his family most valued about him, Sandra revealing remarkable qualities that Angus had not been consciously aware of. I suggested that he might want to consider focussing on himself, and give himself the best chance of recovery, not worry about pleasing others. He is now starting to add up in darts and handle money well and is finally going to the shop on his own. I tentatively suggested Angus talk to his GP about driving again. I asked them to help me to consider how to space our sessions, inviting them to choose the interval that suited them best.

At the end of the conversation, Angus volunteered his view that his speech is getting slowly better. Sandra made the observation that his comprehension has improved enormously in conversation, and I thanked him for being frank with me, that it was good he could express how he had been feeling and that his feelings were entirely understandable. At this point he asked me with a smile what I had planned for this session: we proceeded with single word judgement tasks which he completed rapidly and with success. Boosted by this, he asked for more to practice at home:

- Sentence reading judgments: Angus was able to read, self-correct and re-read accurately the sentences and his judgements of semantic accuracy were 100%. He was pleased with this and reassured about his ability to read.

- Word finding tasks given for him to do if wishes at home. He is using Talkpath app at home.
- Continue with judgements in sessions/ sentence completion and word finding at home
- Started with listening lists, Angus was able to label correctly 100%, but needed some repetitions to hear the word. He could accurately repeat after a pause.
- Reading comprehension – two sentences and answering q's yes vs no. He did very well on this and retained what he had read in order to answer the questions.
- Word finding around a verb – good word retrieval, albeit phonological inaccuracies.

When conversation was self-initiated, Angus could talk about playing golf, for example, in complete, accurate sentences. Reading aloud helped him to access phonology via the orthographic route when semantics to phonology failed. He completed tasks at home with 90% accuracy, and slowly gained confidence, talking more slowly. We worked on some functional tasks such as a TV schedule and written questions with choice of answers, followed by questions about what types of programmes are on and asking what time and channel. Initially he would search randomly for answers and become confused. He then started to develop a strategy for looking for answers more systematically. He started to read aloud accurately after some initial hesitation. Inaccurate stress patterns were hard to correct; however, after a slight distraction, he was able to return to the word and produce it accurately.

We discussed how written information helps with processing. Angus's reading was better than auditory processing, and it slowed him down for spoken output. Angus was using more humour, still feeling extreme fatigue but seeming more optimistic about the future.

The range of further therapy activities included:

- Listening lists – listening only to items presented with semantic distractors and judging whether they belong in the given category.
- Rapid identification of target noun from seven related nouns.
- Sentence formulation with two words, three words and pictures; challenging due to distraction by other items and anxiety about performing well.

- Exercises on the iPad at home, choosing to read some children books, which he is finding easier as practice.
- Newcastle reading 4.1 selection options. Listening to sentence anomalies - needed on occasion to see written form to make decision which he could do easily but not always from auditory signal alone.
- Practice reading aloud to increase OOL-POL process as semantics is relatively strong.
- Reading aloud the articles in 4.1. Used a finger to track words to help to slow him down. In auditory processing he asked for repetition and started to hold on to information he has read quite well. any noise/distraction impacted negatively on his auditory comprehension.
- Synonym judgments
- Newcastle verb comprehension – 31/32
- Newcastle sentence construction C2–1–15. He soon got the hang of this but needed to focus on the action – tended to produce nouns easily but this made it harder to find verb if it wasn't a suitable argument.
- Pictures suggesting SVO: (subject-verb-object). Angus produced a sentence which I wrote for him to check. Some verb errors, some mapping (hanging on the arm = branch) but able to identify and correct well
- Three words suggesting a verb. After two examples Angus grasped the aim of the task and scored 70% in this task – sometimes retrieved noun instead of verb.
- Provided functional reading comprehension tasks e.g., form filling.
- Progressed to harder comprehension passages and proof-reading prepositional errors.
- Reading sentences with verb anomalies – needed prompts to stop himself from going off at tangents.
- Quick fire word finding – 80% wh- words, which shows hugely improved comprehension of wh- structures. Good requests for repetition showing increasing insight.
- Drawing to instruction – concentrate hard, with some error on 3 pieces of information.
- Listening and identifying semantic groups from spoken word lists - 4 words then 5. Marked drop off after 5 but errors were semantically related.
- Watching the news using visual modality only (also for his YouTube videos on art.) This way he can watch news on iPlayer and rewind subtitles if necessary, without the distraction of sound and the auditory processing which he finds most difficult.

- Cuespeak was set up on Angus's iPad with Senfill exercises, word finding quiz and phonology exercises as trialled together in the session. With time and repeated practice, he started to manage phonological tasks as well as comprehension of Wh-sentences, as long as he had the written tabs to support processing sentence meaning. He started to reach targets with greater accuracy, self-correcting his errors, showing greater awareness while talking. The intuitive nature of the app meant that after only a few items Angus could navigate the exercises, hear the words spoken repeatedly, observe a video articulating the word and obtain instant feedback on his responses. The option to use an almost errorless approach to tasks helped to build up his confidence rapidly, leading to greater risk-taking in what he would be prepared to tackle.
- TalkPath News – Angus likes this as he can track the story, as it is read (TV news is overwhelming and subtitles too fast).

Angus reported feeling fitter, and his knees no longer hurting, longer stamina for treadmill and fewer naps in daytime. He could see his speech progressing and could envisage his return to working eventually but said he just hadn't realised it would take so long. (From my perspective being familiar with aphasia, it didn't seem long.) We discussed his progress with speech, reading and comprehension. Sandra was noticing significant improvement and that he was starting to talk to his golfing friends more happily now. We moved to fortnightly sessions with the agreement that we could go back to weekly if needed.

When it became evident that his business would probably fold, Angus began to consider a 'wider' life and started to do more at home. He was teaching himself to paint using YouTube videos, and spending hours at this while Sandra went to work. He worked in the garden, preparing pots for flowers and did some DIY. He planned to work freelance for people eventually.

One day he and Sandra wanted to talk about Angus's sense that some people locally avoid him in the street. We explored the range of possible explanations for this; I had already emphasised the need to make the first move and greet people and Angus carried a stroke association card which explained his aphasia. The discussion concluded with the realisation that prior to his stroke Angus never had a beard and glasses; more often than not, they just weren't recognising him!

Nevertheless, Angus's concern that people might avoid him was tied up in increased awareness of his tendency to get muddled, become verbose and inaccurate when nervous, leading to perseveration of his errors. We explored once more his own auditory processing and self-monitoring skills, and how this might affect his own awareness of accuracy, and under what conditions. I explained that his own self-monitoring is tricky as he has to process his own output auditorily. I drew his attention to that fact that he often self-corrected when he didn't need to, which could lead to further confusion for both parties. Within these conversations I always asked Angus what *his* experience of what I was trying to explain was, whether it was similar or dissimilar and how, in order to ensure that I wasn't making assumptions. The three of us decided that Sandra would start to feed his responses back to him, so that he could start to judge accuracy for himself. Sandra would also encourage Angus to take a risk and talk to people, using his card if necessary.

Angus and Sarah had been talking about having a holiday. Previously Sandra spent a week each year with some girlfriends, but now she was nervous about leaving Angus at home. Angus himself talked about the enormous responsibility Sandra has been carrying, caring for him while also working, and supporting the rest of the family. Angus said, 'she needs a holiday . . . from me'. Sandra reluctantly acknowledged that: 'Angus is very self-contained at home and I don't worry too much but he does become stressed about things if they don't go to plan.' Angus said that he was going to try to address that and call his brother to help if there was a problem: 'After all, he has been absolutely no use to me so far...'

Recently many friends and family had said they couldn't believe how much progress Angus had made recently. Angus wanted to give therapy a break for a while. He wasn't interested in attending the aphasia café, as he knew he couldn't manage a group of more than three people at a time. (Furthermore, unless it was about golfing, it held little interest and he never was one for groups anyway!)

We planned a review session two months from that day. He and Sandra drove to see me. He couldn't believe how fast the two months had gone, and I joked that I wouldn't hold him to continuing therapy. He was enjoying driving now and was playing golf occasionally with a good friend. He had a new puppy which he enjoyed looking after during the day when Sandra was at work. He was meeting new people in walks everyday who spoke to him about the dog. He observed that his anxiety about talking disappeared when the focus was on the dog and not on him and he was managing better. Angus was completing a new painting every day with increasing skill. He was creating and selling planters online and he felt that his understanding was still improving all the time. He still couldn't cope with more than four people in a group and tended to have 1:1 conversations only, but he was content with his day- to-day life now. We ended with a conversation full of humour and optimism, in spite of ongoing struggles with errors from time to time.

Angus was going to continue to practise with Cuespeak and I adjusted some of the exercises for him once more. I offered to do so any time in future if he wanted to call in, or if he wanted to talk anything through. I haven't seen him since, but our last session was a joy to experience.

References

Aphasia United, Best Practice Recommendations. Available at: www.aphasiau nited.org/wp-content/uploads/2016/05/English-Aphasia-United-Best-Practices-Recommendations1.pdf

Asen, E., Tomson, D., Young, V. and Tomson, P. (2004) *Ten Minutes for the Family: Systemic Interventions in Primary Care*. Routledge.

Baker, C., Worrall, L., Rose, M., Hudson, K., Ryan, B. and O'Byrne, L. (2017) A systematic review of rehabilitation interventions to prevent and treat depression in post-stroke aphasia. *Disability and Rehabilitation*.

Carr, A. (1998) Michael White's narrative therapy. *Contemporary Family Therapy*, 20(4): 485–503.

Cecchin, G. (1987) Hypothesizing, circularity, and neutrality revisited: An invitation to curiosity. *Family Process*, 26(4): 405–413.

Cruice, M. Worrall, L. Murison, R. and Hickson, L. (2003) Finding a focus for quality of life with aphasia: social and emotional health, and psychological well-being. *Aphasiology*, 17 4: 333–353.

Doan, R. E. (1998) The king is dead; long live the king: Narrative therapy and practicing what we preach. *Family Process*, 37(3): 379–385.

Ellmo, W., Graser, J., Krchnavek, B., Hauck, K. and Calabrese, D., (1995. Measure of cognitive-linguistic abilities (MCLA). The Speech Bin, Incorporated.

Hackett, M.L., Yapa, C., Parag, V. and Anderson, C.S., 2005. Frequency of depression after stroke: a systematic review of observational studies. *Stroke*, 36(6): 1330–1340.

Hersh, D., Worrall, L., Howe, T., Sherratt, S. and Davidson, B. (2012) SMARTER goal-setting in aphasia rehabilitation. *Aphasiology*, 26(2): 220–233.

House, A., Knapp, P., Bamford, J. and Vail, A., 2001. Mortality at 12 and 24 months after stroke may be associated with depressive symptoms at 1 month. *Stroke*, 32(3): 696–701.

Lanyon, L., Worrall, L. and Rose, M. (2018) What really matters to people with aphasia when it comes to group work? A qualitative investigation of factors impacting participation and integration. *International Journal of Language and Communication Disorders*, May;53(3): 526–541.

Murdock, N.L. (2009) 'Narrative therapy'. In *Theories of Counselling and Psychotherapy: A Case Approach*. Pearson Education, 2nd edition.

NHS Improvement (2011) Psychological care after stroke: Improving stroke services for people with cognitive and mood disorders. NHS Improvement – Stroke.

Pohjasvaara, T., Vataja, R., Leppävuori, A., Kaste, M. and Erkinjuntti, T. (2001) Depression is an independent predictor of poor long-term functional outcome post-stroke. *European Journal of Neurology*, 8(4): 315–319.

Rivett, M. and Street, E. (2009) *Family Therapy: 100 Key Points & Techniques*. Routledge.

Roth, A. and Fonagy, P. (1996) *What Works for Whom? A Critical View of Psychotherapy Research*. Guilford Press.

Springer, L. (2003) 'Reduced Syntax Therapy (REST): A compensatory approach to agrammatism'. In I. Papathanasiou and R. De Bleser (Eds), *The Sciences of Aphasia* (pp. 149–160). Pergamon.

Swain, J. and French, S. (Eds) (2008) *Disability on Equal Terms*. Sage.

Todd, D. and Weatherhead, S. (Eds) (2018) *Narrative Approaches to Brain Injury*. Routledge.

White, M. (1998) August. Narrative therapy. In workshop presented at Narrative Therapy Intensive Training.

White, M., Wijaya, M., White, M.K. and Epston, D. (1990). *Narrative Means to Therapeutic Ends*. W. W. Norton.

Worrall, L. (2019) The seven habits of highly effective aphasia therapists: The perspective of people living with aphasia. *International Journal of Speech-Language Pathology*, 21(5): 438–447.

Worrall, L. E., Hudson, K., Khan, A., Ryan, B. and Simmons-Mackie, N. (2016) Determinants of living well with aphasia in the first year poststroke: A prospective cohort study. *Archives of Physical Medicine and Rehabilitation*, 98(2): 235–240.

Worrall, L., Sherratt, S., Rogers, P., Howe, T., Hersh, D., Ferguson, A. and Davidson, B. (2011) What people with aphasia want: Their goals according to the ICF. *Aphasiology*, 25(3): 309–322.

Zimmerman, J. L. and Dickerson, V. C. (2001) 'Narrative therapy'. In R. Corsini (Ed.), *Handbook of Innovative Psychotherapies* (pp. 415–426). John Wiley & Sons.

9 | Final thoughts

Never has the situation been more challenging for people with aphasia than during the global pandemic of the last year. Separated from family and loved ones, those who need care and rehabilitation have endured even greater isolation than in usual times. Therapists have been unable to work so closely with family and carers to demonstrate techniques, or even to prioritise communication assessments and therapy. As I write, Paddy has been on a neurology ward for two weeks, after a second bleed at the age of 60. His son has been told only that he is unable to speak, and that the prognosis is poor. He already had moderate aphasia and is getting increasingly agitated, but a referral for an aphasia assessment from the SLT department just a few steps away has not been made. Is there not a more urgent time for establishing how much Paddy understands, and in what modalities (e.g., visual or auditory), so that his son can know how to communicate with him as he approaches what is quite likely to be a premature end to his life? Why don't medical staff know when to refer for communication assessment and why understanding is not the same as speaking?

Families have been unable to reassure and support the PWA with their familiarity and their shared stories during the pandemic. We know that people with significant cognitive deficits can still preserve a construct of self and that carers play an important role in maintaining both positive selfhood for that person and in maintaining family discourse. Prohibited contact with family over the last year has severely limited this.

Families or close social networks

Regardless of the pandemic, indeed prior to that, relatives of PWA often said that how individuals in the multidisciplinary rehabilitation team choose to

DOI: 10.4324/9781003178613-9

do their jobs, is what makes the difference to them and their loved one with aphasia. It seems tragic to me that families feel it is down to sheer chance whether the therapist they encounter 'chooses' to work in a particular way. I find it unacceptable that people with aphasia in our society, some of the most vulnerable people there are if they cannot communicate, do not routinely have access to good quality aphasia therapy.

Families need to be recognised, with their burden of caring, financial, and many other roles, their loneliness and frustration. Medical focus is normally on the PWA, and partners put themselves last. Their exhaustion and distress will of course affect the PWA, but also others in the wider family network and this comes back to affect the PWA.

Sometimes the PWA expects to be treated as a priority in the longer term, making it harder for families to return to a sense of normal functioning again. There may be children to care for too, or even elderly parents. Spouses may feel guilty for feeling annoyed and frustrated and children may even hear their parent wishing they had died. Family members all deal differently with the scenario that plays out, some coping in the early stage, others at a later stage.

Family (or other close social network) is key, and by working systemically, from a community base and in the context of people's lives, we can begin to offer truly holistic rehabilitation to the PWA and, crucially, to their family or close network. Asking for help from friends and relatives is very hard; families want to protect their privacy and therapists need to be more skilled in how they respect and interact with the family context as a whole. To recall Desmond Tutu, 'a person is not basically an independent, solitary entity. A person is human precisely in being enveloped in the community of other human beings, in being caught up in the bundle of life. To be . . . is to participate' (Krog 1998).

Acquiring aphasia can often mean losing hope. People working with aphasia need to embrace hope for the PWA and for their family too, whether they are doctors, nurses or therapists. An authentic sense of hope can be engendered through a systemic approach to therapeutic intervention. As Feldman and Snyder (2005) explain; 'Hope is something we do with others. Hope is too important—its effects on body and soul too significant—to be left to individuals alone. Hope must be the responsibility of the community. Where this is so, and when this is so, there will be a sense of wonder, which has been called the abyss where radical amazement occurs . . . . Ours. Together. With hope'.

Hilari et al (2021) report 'There is pressing need to systematically evaluate interventions to improve wellbeing for people with aphasia.' They say that 'Interventions for people with aphasia with no/mild mood problems that avert some of the long-term psychological consequences of stroke may prevent the need for more complex and costly psychological therapies'. They suggest peer-befriending as one solution. In my experience, even mild mood problems are more complex than this, and it takes skilled therapeutic support to address this right from the early stages of aphasia. Concentrating on treating the mood of the individual client is not sufficient in addressing quality of life challenges in aphasia; the wider system is key. 'Costly and complex psychological therapies' don't ever happen, as far as I am aware, even when the mood problems are severe. The PWA's silence precludes a demand for such a service. The reality is that nobody offers psychological therapy to the person with severe aphasia: there is resounding silence in relation to this population. Instead, this person has their behaviours 'managed' in the long term by carers with inadequate training.

Limited experience of aphasia by an SLT does not prevent them from being recruited to work in a complex brain injury rehabilitation setting currently, as long as they have the dysphagia experience that will protect the organisation from litigation. I have seen this myself recently. After all, how many applicants for these roles can demonstrate extensive experience in this field and what alternative does the employer have?

Whether a client has the mental capacity to say where they want to live and who cares for them, and be supported to express such choices, seems to be of lesser importance to organisations. Why is an aphasia therapist still not involved in each and every assessment of mental capacity of the person with aphasia? The skilled therapist will also be aware, that in privileging the voice and independence of the PWA they must not overlook their vulnerability and need for protection; a very fine balance to try to achieve. I am still stumbling across mental capacity oversights where PWA are concerned, despite widespread mandatory training in the NHS on the Mental Capacity Act of 2005. There is still so much difference in the quality of aphasia knowledge and skills training that students emerge with into the workplace, and in the knowledge they encounter when they get there.

A new toolkit

Is it time to review the aphasia components of undergraduate training? I frequently wonder whether aphasia should be a distinct module with specific competencies for development of specialism. Aphasia often feels like the poor relation in SLT work, and community SLT is seen as the poor relation in SLT work with the adult health population. This is evident in the recruitment bias towards acute settings and dysphagia, and in the impossible demands often placed on a community therapist. Calling something supported conversation sounds like a simple solution to a challenging problem. It is not. The term alone doesn't fully define it, or mean it is delivered skilfully, or even prove that the PWA is helped by it. Knowing how to be an aphasia therapist, in my view, takes an alternative way of seeing things, tenacity, and a great deal of practice. Intrinsic day to day modelling, by aphasia therapists, in hospital settings, and in the community is the best way to train others, but such therapists have to be present, 'on the ground', in these places. In the future I wonder whether in-reach by the community aphasia specialist who knows what community life holds, and before the patient leaves hospital, is a better way forward for aphasia families.

The aphasia therapist's toolkit might well include the full range of aphasia interventions, but also many of the systemic techniques outlined so far in this book.

- We would do well to shift the balance of power, to one that is about collaboration as has been discussed widely in this book.
- We could shift from 'deficit' to 'appreciative' language. Gergen (1999) has shown that our 'normal' language has a large proportion of expressions and vocabulary that focus on what is missing, what is wrong, and what can't be done. Deborah Tannen (2007) describes our culture as one in which the default option is argument and conflict rather than cooperation and dialogue. However, as we have seen, social realities can be powerfully impacted if people's lives are described appreciatively and with hope. Viktor Frankl, a Holocaust survivor and psychiatrist from Vienna, refers to the ability to maintain hope and find meaning in crisis as tragic optimism, or 'the human capacity to creatively turn life's negative aspects into something positive or constructive' (Frankl 1985).
- Systemic thinking does not view change as a fixed event. Rather, it holds a different meaning for each person. Conversations must start with what the person understands about what has happened to them; listening to what they know is an important first step, otherwise the information you present to them might as well just dangle in mid-air, it can't connect to anything that is already 'real' for them.

- When a survey asked people, who had a stroke what was most important to them in those early days, the most common answer was 'kindness' and understanding; not testing, advice, prognosis, medication and all the other things we throw at patients in our medicalised approach to treatment. As Plato once said (427–347 BC), 'If you want to heal the body, you must first heal the mind.'

- We might move away from biomedical diagnoses in aphasia therapy; diagnoses reduce complexity, are not balanced enough and can shut down creativity.

- Dichotomies that are often presented in discussions around aphasia are shown actually not to be such when a systemic view is adopted. Rather, a fluid view of ideas being 'both...and...' may be more helpful to ourselves as well as those we work with.

- Systemic thinking holds the view that change is more likely to be maintained if internally driven. If the client has a sense of having drawn on their own resources and knowledge it increases the possibility, they will look to themselves to deal with future challenges.

- Circular questioning can be powerful with other family members present. For example, by asking Jane with aphasia how she thinks John's life has changed, it was revealed that he is suffering more than she is, because she forgets things so easily.

- Let us challenge the notion of 'plateau'. Individuals have highly variable patterns of recovery which cannot be predicted early on in the rehabilitation process.

- We could become less certain of the positions we hold. When we become less certain of the positions we hold, we are more likely to become receptive to other possibilities, other meanings we might put to events. If we can become more open to the possible influence of other perspectives, we open up space for other views to be stated and heard (Mason 1992, 2002, 2009).

- Let us think about lifecycles – be overt about transgenerational themes, patterns and beliefs in families. Do some of these alter now aphasia is in your life, or do you resolutely hold on to them and resist 'giving in' to them?

To these, I would add maxims for interactions as suggested by Pearce and Pearce (2004), with the proviso that they are incorporated into training within a new systemic mindset around aphasia therapy:

- Treat all stories, your own as well as others, as incomplete, unfinished, biased, and inconsistent.
- Treat your own stories as 'local', dependent on your own perspective, history, and purposes.
- Treat stories that differ from your own as 'valid' within the framework of the other person's perspective, history, and purposes.
- Be curious about other people's stories.
- Be aware that you are participating in a multi-turn process.
- Be aware that you are part of, but only part of, a multi-person process.
- Be mindful that this process involves reciprocally responding to and eliciting responses from other people.
- Be mindful that this process creates the social world in which we all live.

Above all, we have to remember that, however much we work, learn and study, and regardless of how much clinical experience we might have, 'human knowledge is never contained in one person. It grows from the relationships we create between each other and the world and still it is never complete' (Kalanithi 2016).

References

Feldman, D. B. and Snyder, C. R. (2005) Hope and the meaningful life: Theoretical and empirical associations between goal-directed thinking and life meaning. *Journal of Social and Clinical Psychology*, 24(3): 401–421.

Frankl, V. E. (1985) *Man's Search for Meaning*. Simon and Schuster.

Gergen, K. J. (1999) *An Invitation to Social Construction*. Sage.

Hilari, K., Behn, N., James, K., Northcott, S., Marshall, J., Thomas, S., Simpson, A., Moss, B., Flood, C., McVicker, S. and Goldsmith, K., 2021. Supporting wellbeing through peer-befriending (SUPERB) for people with aphasia: A feasibility randomised controlled trial. *Clinical Rehabilitation*, 35(8). doi:10.1177/0269215521995671

Kalanithi, P. (2016) *When Breath Becomes Air*. Random House.

Krog, A., 1998. The Truth and Reconciliation Commission: a national ritual? *Missionalia: Southern African Journal of Mission Studies*, 26(1): 5–16.

Mason, B. (1993) Towards positions of safe uncertainty, *Human Systems: The Journal of Systemic Consultation and Management*, 4: 189–200.

Pearce, W.B. and Pearce, K.A. (2004) 'Taking a communication perspective on dialogue'. In R. Anderson, L. Baxter and K. N. Cissna (Eds), *Dialogue: Theorizing Difference in communication Studies* (pp. 39–56). Sage.

Tannen, D. (2007) *Talking Voices: Repetition, Dialogue, and Imagery in Conversational Discourse* (Vol. 26). Cambridge University Press.

Index

CPSIA information can be obtained
at www.ICGtesting.com
Printed in the USA
LVHW112048141221
706193LV00009B/302

9 781032 014371